Take Your Oxygen First

Praise for *Take Your Oxygen First*

"Take Your Oxygen First is a personal, frank and touching look inside a family's journey with Alzheimer's disease. But even more importantly, it is a clear guidebook to better understanding the disease and its phases, written in language that is understood by all. The book is filled with specific, practical reminders and directions for family caregivers. The loving message throughout is that, in order to best care for the person you love, you have to first care for yourself."

CHERYL PHILLIPS, M.D., PRESIDENT, AMERICAN GERIATRICS SOCIETY

"Dr. Jamie Huysman, Dr. Rosemary Laird and Leeza Gibbons and family have created an indispensable workbook that all family caregivers must make sure they keep on their nightstand and read the first thing in the morning and the last thing at night."

GARY EDWARD BARG, EDITOR-IN-CHIEF, *Today's Caregiver Magazine*

"Take Your Oxygen First gives both the science and the personal experiences of Leeza Gibbons and her family that every Alzheimer's caregiver will benefit from."

Preserving Your Memory Magazine

"Getting older is not always easy, especially when it involves caring for a loved one with Alzheimer's disease. The physical and emotional toll on caregivers can be profound. Paradoxically, by neglecting their own health, caregivers are more likely to suffer depression, anxiety, insomnia, and other illnesses, thus becoming less effective at caring for their loved one. If you are a caregiver, *Take Your Oxygen First* is a must-read. By sharing in Leeza Gibbons' journey of caring for her mother with Alzheimer's disease, you will learn the importance of caring for yourself first. This book can be your "field manual," providing you with practical guidance on leading a life of wholeness and fulfillment while shouldering the responsibilities of a caregiver."

KEVIN W. O'NEIL, M.D., FACP, MEDICAL DIRECTOR, BROOKDALE SENIOR LIVING

Take Your
Oxygen First

PROTECTING YOUR HEALTH *and*

HAPPINESS WHILE CARING *for*

a LOVED ONE *with* MEMORY LOSS

Leeza Gibbons

James Huysman, PsyD, LCSW

Rosemary DeAngelis Laird, M.D.

LACHANCE PUBLISHING ▪ NEW YORK

ISBN: 9781934184202

Edited by Victor Starsia and Richard Day Gore

Cover and Interior Design by Stewart A. Williams

Library of Congress Control Number: 2008939968

Publisher: LaChance Publishing, LLC
120 Bond Street
Brooklyn, NY 11217
www.lachancepublishing.com

Distributor:Independent Publishers Group
814 North Franklin Street
Chicago, IL 60610
www.ipgbook.com

This book is available at special discounts for bulk purchases for sales
promotions and premiums. Special editions, including personalized cov-
ers, excerpts, and corporate imprints can be created in large quantities
for special needs. For more information, please write to LaChance Publishing, LLC, 120 Bond Street, Brooklyn, NY 11217 or email at info@

*C*hances are that everyone who reads this book has had the experience of waking up one day and asking themselves, "how am I going to do this?" When your chance at "happily ever after" fades in the face of the new demands placed upon you, courage is not an option. No one orders up a life as a caregiver, but being one can be the most direct path to knowing who you really are.

This book is a love letter and a lifeline to all of those caregivers who have ever felt lost and afraid. We have learned so much about grace and goodness from all the caregivers we have had the pleasure to know and work with all over the country, and we dedicate this book to each of you, and to all of the families who look down a long tunnel and fail to see any light at all yet manage to hope and believe and wake up one more day to do it all over again.

This book is also dedicated to Jean Dyson Gibbons, who taught her family how to make their lives stand for something, and to never look down on anyone unless they were reaching to lift them up. Her voice and life stands for the empowerment she never quite found for herself but managed somehow to give to her family.

Contents

PART II: *Caring For the Caregiver's Body*

PART III: *Caring for the Caregiver's Mind*

Foreword

In 2001 we had my old friend Nancy Reagan on *Larry King Live* for the occasion of President Reagan's 90th birthday. Not long before, the President had announced to the country his diagnosis with Alzheimer's disease. That announcement went a long way towards raising public awareness of the disorder, both in this country and around the world.

Anyone who knows anything about Alzheimer's disease knows how difficult it is giving constant care to someone with this terrible illness. I asked Nancy during that interview what she felt was the most difficult part about having a loved one living with this disease, thinking that she would describe the physical toll that it took on her beloved husband and on his family. She surprised me when she said the hardest part about it was that she was no longer able to share with her him all of the wonderful memories of the extraordinary life they had lived together. I thought to myself, how different this disease is from every other, how much more terrible it is in some ways, that it can take the person you love from you long before that person leaves this earth. How hard it must be on the family, who might live for many years with a person whose essence is lost piece by piece.

In 2005, I heard from another good friend of mine that this disease had taken yet another person. Anyone who has met Leeza Gibbons knows that she is one of those people who lights up a room as soon as she walks in. A terrific personality combined with great intelligence and a great beauty as well, Leeza is a human hurricane of activity. From her success on radio and television to her innovative approach to the business of business, she has been one of the few people to whom I have turned to guest host my show, because I know Leeza puts her heart and soul into everything she does. We have known each other for many years, and our kids, my Chance and her Nathan, have faced off in many a Little League game.

My heart went out to her as she explained that her mother, Gloria Jean, who had been diagnosed with Alzheimer's disease over a decade before, was then in the end stages of the disease. As this insidious "thief of memories" stole Gloria Jean from her family, she explained, it also created tremendous personal challenges for all those around her. Some years before, Leeza told me of her idea to start a foundation, in memory of her mother, that would be dedicated to helping all of those giving care to a person suffering from Alzheimer's disease and other memory loss disorders. I offered my help and since then, the Leeza Gibbons Memory Foundation has grown from a single community center helping caregivers living in Los Angeles to a network of centers known as Leeza's Place, helping people help themselves at locations around the country.

For Leeza, there is only one way to move, and that is forward. I know she sees the success of Leeza's Place as another opportunity to reach many more caregivers around the country. Leeza and her co-authors have now distilled all of the advice and support they give to caregivers at Leeza's Place into this wonderful book. Yes, *Take Your Oxygen First* is filled with great information about Alzheimer's disease and other memory loss disorders, and the most effective ways a caregiver can take care of him or herself in order to give the best care possible to a loved one. But it is much more. Leeza and her entire family, from young Nathan to Leeza's dad Carlos, have opened up their hearts in the most candid and courageous way. They tell the sometimes painful, other times joyous story of life with Gloria Jean and the challenges the family faced in struggling with this illness. I learned things I never knew about my dear friend Leeza, but I learned much more: I also learned how strong the human spirit can be in the face of grave adversity.

In my years hosting *Larry King Live*, I've interviewed many individuals who have faced chronic and life threatening illnesses: the Reagans, Lance Armstrong, Michael J. Fox, Mohammed Ali, Dana and Christopher Reeve, and more. In both my public and private conversations with these people, one theme has regularly emerged—that there were moments when they were confronted with a harsh diagnosis and did not know where to turn for information and support. For those facing the daunting challenges of caring for someone with a memory loss disorder, that vacuum is eloquently filled by Leeza, her co-authors, and the Gibbons family with *Take Your Oxygen First*. If there is one thing every reader will gain from this book, it is the message of hope that pervades every page. For those who are just starting out on the journey of caring for a loved one and for those already caught up in its tremendous burdens, seeing that light at the end of the tunnel can seem all but impossible. I was surprised and gratified to learn that despite the nature of this terrible illness, *Take Your Oxygen First* shows caregivers that the act of giving care can actually be a life sustaining and empowering experience for them, for their families and for their loved one as well.

—*Larry King*

My Family – And Yours

In my business, I'm used to getting requests for interviews. They usually aren't personal; most often I'm asked to talk about someone who has appeared on my show. But the call I got from *People Magazine* when I was producing and hosting my daily talk show *Leeza* was different. The *People* reporter didn't want to talk about one of my guests. He wanted me to talk about my mother. Only 63, she'd just been diagnosed with Alzheimer's disease. News travels fast in my business, and the news was out that Mom was sick. My family barely had a chance to deal with this news privately, now we had to decide how to deal with it publicly.

My family is the great blessing of my life. We're all wildly different but wonderfully close, and at the center of it all was my mom, Gloria Jean Dyson Gibbons, Jean to her friends, "J.G." to her grandkids. When *People* made its request for a story, I went to Mom, my dad, Carlos, Sr., my sister, Cammy, my sister-in-law, Anne Marie and my brother, Carlos, Jr. and asked how they felt about a story on Mom appearing in a national magazine. Mom didn't hesitate, not for a second. She gave us our marching orders. She made the whole family promise that we would do whatever we could to tell her story, in the hope that it would in some way help the many millions of people who were going through what our family was now facing. "Make it count," she said. We promised to do just that, and participating in the *People* story would be the first step in keeping our promise to Mom, a promise we continue to honor with this book.

She was living at home at the time, being cared for by my Dad but still very much aware of what was going on. I helped her pick out some nice clothes and we did her makeup as best we could. She was serene that day; her smile was clear and there was a softness about her. The *People* reporter and photographer were very kind and put Mom at ease. My favorite picture from that shoot was of her and me sitting on the hammock in the yard by the lake we called "Golden Pond." I had my arms wrapped around her and we were sharing a laugh. It was a bittersweet moment, because I knew connecting with her like that wouldn't be possible for much longer. A flood of memories washed over me, memories that seemed more precious than ever, because I knew Mom's own memories were already fading away, stolen by Alzheimer's disease.

I've always been so proud of my mom. A true "steel magnolia," she stood up for herself all of her life, overcoming the challenges of being a small town girl with a high school education in a changing world, born into a generation of women who were pretty much seen and not heard. She brought that same determination to her struggle with Alzheimer's disease. But there was more than just her strong personality pushing Mom to tell her story, to make sure she was heard. You see, her mother, Marie Dyson, suffered from the same disease.

Granny was the most tender soul I have ever known. She was plump with an ample bosom and it all got moving when she laughed, which was often. She was born in Clarendon County in South Carolina and lived there until she died. Her husband, my grandfather, who died at a very young age, was the one true love of her life. Granny never remarried, but she was never bitter. Her life as a single woman for so many years made her strong, and she never shied away from an opportunity to open her heart and her home to others. My fondest memories of Granny are of spending time with her in her kitchen. She used to make the best homemade biscuits from scratch and, when they were fresh out of the oven, she would let us kids pop our thumbs into the side of each biscuit to make a well which she would fill with Cane Patch syrup, so sweet it would rot your teeth with the first bite. As kids, we knew that we'd never have a better friend or a stronger ally than Granny. She fed our bodies with good home cooking and our hearts with love, and she was always on our side.

Ironically, one of the first signs of Granny's dementia appeared while we were together in her kitchen. Granny had made biscuits, but she couldn't find them. When she opened the oven and it was empty, I saw the look on her face and knew something was wrong. She finally found the baking sheet full of biscuits in a dresser drawer in her bedroom. It wasn't long before the disease took hold of Granny. Mom spent years caring for Granny, who would, soon after that day in the kitchen, begin to forget her daughter. .

Mom grew up a tomboy but became sort of a cross between Jackie Onassis, Cher and June Cleaver, with each of the personalities competing for dominance. I remember watching Mom get all dolled up for a night out with Dad. She used to keep her hair platinum blonde and wore a "fall", a hairpiece that she would pile high on her head and sometimes set off with an honest-to-goodness tiara, and would finish it all off with a splash of her favorite perfume, Norell. She was funny and free-spirited, but serious about boundaries for her kids, and she always insisted on manners and respect. One summer at Myrtle Beach, Mom walked into the living room of the big vacation house where all of us teenagers were staying and caught me on the sofa kissing my boyfriend. "Oh my goodness, let's call the paramedics," Mom exclaimed. "Leeza has passed out and Billy is giving her C.P.R." Often on sleepovers, Mom would stay up in the kitchen talking with my friends long after I had gone to bed. Her energy was young and boundless.

Mom was quick to support and slow to judge. Like every little girl at some time in their lives, I used to wonder, "Am I smart enough, strong enough, pretty enough?" When I was in grade school there was a talent show and all of my friends were ready to dazzle with their piano playing, their dancing, singing, or crocheting. Everybody had a talent but me. I had nothing, at least nothing I wanted to share. Mom was sympathetic to my tears but she put an end to my whining by saying, "You shush up, Leeza Kim, you do have a talent, you're a story teller, and you're gonna stand up there and tell the story of your life." I don't know how she pulled that out of thin air, but I believed her. Ever since, being a storyteller has been how I define myself.

Daddy is a "life of the party" kind of man, at least that's the way I think of him. If you see a gathering of people in a crowded room, chances are they'll be worshipping at the feet of Carlos, Sr. Truly, all the world's a stage for Daddy. He can whip up a piece of prose in less than five minutes and rhyming poetry quicker than that. He'll recite at the drop of a hat, to almost anyone. When we were growing up, Dad used to make a lot of speeches and public appearances, first as a school principal, then as the Chief Supervisor of Education for South Carolina. He used to keep a "joke file": a box of one-liners and stories sure to crack up his audience that he always tried out on the family first. I was always the most willing participant and would laugh the loudest and longest at anything Daddy said. When the jokes were what Mom would call "in bad taste", Dad and I would just go to another room, where he would deliver the punch lines and I would supply the laughter while Mom rolled her eyes in mock disapproval.

He was always serious, though, about the need to create change and to champion the underdog. I learned much of my compassion and leadership from watching Dad run for political office. After he was elected Chief Supervisor of Education he ran twice for State Superintendent of Education. My time with Dad "stumping" throughout South Carolina was one of the experiences that informed my beliefs the most. I gained respect for the power to touch a life by listening and taking action. Mostly, though, I learned an appreciation for a system of democracy that allows us to speak our minds, vote for our choice and still complain about it later. Daddy always believed in the system and when I looked at the pictures we had of him with John Kennedy and Lyndon Johnson and a score of local political dignitaries, I believed in it too. But despite his public life, when I think of Daddy, the image that most often comes to mind is of him with a fishing pole in hand, usually with his shirt off and wearing some goofy hat, all alone on his dock at the water's edge.

Growing up, I was lucky to have the best brother and sister I could ever want. To this day, my older brother Carlos is the one of the few people I know who can always crack me up. When we were kids, our very similar spirits expressed themselves in different ways. He played in the high school marching band and I was head cheerleader. He collected every *National Geographic* and *Mad Magazine* he ever read (I think he still has them!), while I collected experiences. Carl was the kind of kid who could take one of those standardized tests in a gymnasium full of students and finish early with the highest score. My brother always seemed to do everything right. It was no surprise to any of us that he became an attorney; he is, after all, a Virgo, and order and control are embedded in his core! But also, I think, he entered the profession because of his belief that everyone deserves a chance and he is most happy when he is able to help. But for as hard as he works, Carl never misses an opportunity to play. He has had the same friends for life and is one of the most loyal people you could ever know.

I will always love my brother for one more thing he did just right: marrying Anne Marie Richardson. My sister-in-law is an absolute angel on earth, and my sister Cammy and I have loved Anne Marie since the day we met her. She is as stunningly beautiful now as she was as a young bride, with porcelain skin and the most delicate features. Perfect. Think of the person you feel safest with, the one who could talk you off the ledge, praise you for the smallest thing and make you believe that everything is going to be O.K. That's Anne Marie. In fact, one of the funniest stories during Mom's decline is when Mom was on a tirade, yelling at Cammy and calling her a "witch" (the disease often brings on cursing that comes out of nowhere). She said I was one too. Cammy then asked, "Well if Leeza and I are witches, what is Anne Marie?" "She's the *perfect* witch!" Mom replied. Thank God I had her, my "other sister", to be the center of the see-saw when Mom was diagnosed. Anne Marie was tireless in her efforts in coming up with a plan to care for Mom, because that's what she does best. She was the person I turned to for resources in South Carolina to help Mom while I was living 3,000 miles away in California.

Anne Marie is our soul sister, who inspires us with her sheer goodness and willingness to do whatever is necessary to make life better, safer, richer, and more memorable. She is tough as nails, a characteristic that was fine-tuned after her daughter Taylor was diagnosed with juvenile diabetes. Anne Marie's kindness during our difficult time was unforgettable, but then again, her kindness is legendary in South Carolina and her dogged dedication to charitable causes has moved mountains. My mom called her daughter, Cammy and I call her sister and everyone calls her friend. She makes the journey a little less lonely for all of us.

And then there is my kid sister Cammy, probably the coolest

person I know. She is the free spirit of the family, and her window on the world is stained glass sprinkled with fairy dust. I must have heard Mom say a thousand times that "Cam dances to the beat of a different drummer!" It's true. Cammy will sing opera at the top of her lungs and her young son Blake chimes right in. They have a song for everything and Cam would much rather play in Blake's tree house than be the one to impose discipline. It's her life without boundaries that makes her so unique and so loveable. She embraces people that others would not, and the more offbeat they are the better, as far as she is concerned. Cammy and I became close as adults and we are now the best of friends. She instinctively knows when to call and can always tell what is going on in my life. I'm pretty sure she's psychic; she did study Wicca and knows how to read tarot cards! She has always thought that I was too careful with my words and withholding of my deepest emotions (in this book you'll read how this can be especially bad for you as a caregiver). I remember the first time as an adult that I truly yelled at her. I was screaming at the top of my lungs, just letting her have it about something. She smiled and hugged me and said, "Sis, I'm so proud of you, you're really mad! You love me enough to yell at me!"

Being almost eight years younger than me and ten years behind my brother, Cammy had a different relationship with our parents and with Mom especially. They were more like sisters or friends. They both believed in fairies and magic but mostly, they believed in each other. As you will read, Cammy was the one who moved her life back home to South Carolina to be there for Dad as Mom declined. But we all know you can't go home again, especially when your Mom isn't there. My sister initially went to a pretty dark place and there were times when sweet Cammy (like all of us) would face days full of pain and depression. But we have held each other up and lifted each other's spirits though it all. I would do anything for her and I know she feels the same.

You may have experienced that dark place, and your journey with this dreaded disease may have started as my family's did. We were all gathered at the doctor's office while Mom took a "cognitive functioning test" that would eventually result in her diagnosis with Alzheimer's disease. No one said anything. We didn't have to. We knew. Alzheimer's had caught my family in its grip again. It was heartbreaking to think that Mom would not be able to recall all the stories and events that had made her so strong, that her southern charm and outgoing personality would fade and ultimately disappear. The paradise that had been our lives until then was over. Now we had to begin the process of letting go of Mom.

Nancy Reagan was right when she said that this disease is "the longest goodbye." It's death in slow motion. And not just for the person who has the disease. As a family assuming the role of caregivers, we began to experience, as millions of other caregivers do, a situation that can utterly consume the lives and well being of the people giving care, just as the disorder consumes its victim. We were so overwhelmed that we fumbled through the process almost numb, without a lifeline. But as time passed, we found that each of our different strengths emerged and together as a family we did the best we could possibly do for Mom. My father became a loving caregiver, faithful fundraiser and vigilant fighter. My sister, brother and sister-in-law became soldiers in the same army fighting this disease, spurred on by my mother's courageous insistence that we use her illness as the impetus to inform, educate and advocate, politically and clinically, for others who are suffering in silence—and that includes the families of the people with the disorder. People like you, who may be struggling to maintain your own life and sense of self as you face the challenges of your loved one's illness.

As I've watched this "thief of life and memories" take so much, my desire to help others has grown. When Jamie Huysman (our Executive Director and my good friend) and I founded The Leeza Gibbons Memory Foundation, my dream was to offer a safe setting for families who are dealing with loved ones diagnosed with a memory disorder or any chronic illness or disease. We now offer Leeza's Place, community-based centers offering free services for caregivers and for the newly diagnosed. Leeza's Place is meant to be an oasis where these individuals and families can gather their strength and make a plan. They can connect with others, find resources and encouragement for their difficult work, and become empowered to maintain joy in their own lives even while dealing with a devastating illness. The number of Leeza's Place locations is growing, and we are on our way to reaching our goal of having a Leeza's place in every state.

In the meantime, we've learned a great deal about the burdens faced by so many in caring for a loved one with memory loss, both through the experience of my own family and through the work we've done with so many caregivers, and the families of caregivers, around the country. We want to share these experiences with you, and this book is meant to benefit those of you who are out there braving the challenges of caregiving. In *Take Your Oxygen First*, my family and I open our hearts and share our experiences giving care to Jean—experiences that may mirror your own as you give care to a loved one with a memory loss disorder. Our wonderful co-authors, Jamie Huysman and Dr. Rosemary DeAngelis Laird, contribute their knowledge to provide you with valuable information and advice that they give to caregivers who visit us at Leeza's Place every day. Consider this book to be a visit to Leeza's Place! Just as we would do if you walked in our doors, with *Take Your Oxygen First* we hope to empower you, the caregiver, to enhance your self esteem, reduce your stress, and ultimately improve the quality of your life.

In these pages you'll hear from Dad and Cammy, Anne Marie, Carlos and me as we share our heartfelt and honest experiences of caregiving for Jean. You'll also hear from our kids. At the Memory Foundation we feel that children are all too often left out of the caregiving process, and their exclusion creates an emotional distance between them and the person with a memory loss disorder. I didn't want that to happen with my own children, Lexi, Troy and Nathan, and their closeness to their grandmother has been the inspiration behind many of our programs to keep the generations together during these difficult times. They have many thoughts to share about their "J.G.," and you'll find them in *Take Your Oxygen First*, together with words from their cousins, Kelly and Taylor, my brother Carlos and Anne Marie's kids, and even Cammy's 7 year-old Blake.

We are a family, related by blood, bonded by emotion and blessed by deep commitment to one another. We share our story because we hope it can help, because people are hurting and because Mom asked us to. Like so many of you, while we wait for a miracle, we learn, we fight, we push for a cure and we lean on each other for strength. Our mission began with our commitment to bare our souls in that *People Magazine* article, when Mom told us to tell our story and "make it count." I will always remember the warm and protective hug I gave Mom when the photographer from the magazine took our picture that crisp fall day. It was the same kind she had given me so many times in my life when I needed one the most. That picture is on the cover of this book.

In loving memory of my mother Jean Gibbons, we all invite you to share her story—our story—in the hope that you can achieve a better, healthier and more joyful life.

—Leeza

About Leeza's Place

Leeza's Place serves as an emotional oasis for caregivers who need a place to stop and take a breath from their busy lives, to figure out where they stand and where they are headed and as a place where caregivers can connect with the resources that are vital to the physical, emotional and spiritual support of their loved ones and themselves. In the safe, intimate living room setting of Leeza's Place, caregivers can get educated, become empowered and find renewed energy for the long haul of caring for a loved one with a memory loss disorder.

Whether someone is new to the process and needs more information about their disorder, or is a "veteran" caregiver looking for a support group, at Leeza's Place, specially trained "Leeza Care Advocates" help caregivers tap into the specific resources they need.

Each Leeza's Place features a community based Memory Media Center that provides current information about Alzheimer's disease and other memory disorders and includes literature, video and audio tapes, CD's, books and computer stations with Internet access. Visitors can view the materials onsite or check them out to use at home.

Leeza's Place also offers workshops and classes in subjects ranging from Reiki therapy to the legal issues that arise out of a diagnosis of a memory loss disorder,. Most locations offer Memory Screenings, which test memory, language skills, thinking ability and other intellectual functions for the purpose of encouraging early diagnoses and early medical intervention for memory disorders.

When their loved ones have passed on, many caregivers frequently find it helpful to share their expertise and experiences with others facing similar situations. The Leeza's Place Mentoring Program connects veteran caregivers with those new to the process. Those who are just beginning on their caregiving journey are blessed with the wisdom and understanding a mentor like this can bring.

Each Leeza's Place is partnered with a local community health-care system that provides caregivers and their loved ones access to local health and support programs through voluntary organizations, religious groups, for profit, not-for-profit, and governmental agencies.

Leeza's Place was designed to ensure that anyone experiencing what the Gibbons family encountered has access to supportive environments promoting education, empowerment and energy for the journey ahead. For more information on Leeza's Place, please visit www.leezasplace.org.

Acknowledgements

Just saying "thank you" seems pitifully inadequate when it comes to acknowledging the people who have come together to create this book. At the center of it all is my mother, who even in death has managed to offer lessons and extend love that binds us eternally. I am in awe of my family, which has risen to every occasion to share what they know and feel to make it better for someone else. Thanks to my father, Carlos Gibbons, Sr. for inspiring me to believe in my capacity to create change. Dad, Carl, Cam and Anne Marie; I am blessed and privileged to share a name and a life with each of you. You have been the calm eye in my storm of doubt and through your love and faith you have reminded me of what is possible. To my darling children Lexi, Troy and Nathan, you are the heart and soul of everything I do and the reason for every breath I take. Thank you for loving me through my attempts to make it all matter more. To my nieces Taylor and Kelly and my nephew Blake, thanks for reminding me not to take myself all that seriously!

My deep gratitude to Bobby Xydis for his support, reminders, advice, hand-holding and sometimes tough love! Many thanks as well to Vincent Arcuri, Abraham O'Campo and Cheri Ingram, who each in their own way helped me to find purpose from pain. No one is more fortunate than me to be blessed with such incredible friends.

The Leeza Gibbons Memory Foundation would not exist without Dr. Jamie Huysman. Not only was he a valued (and my favorite) guest on my talk show, he became a close friend and mentor. It was Jamie's gentle guidance and his never-ending love and energy that made our foundation and Leeza's Place a reality. I'm grateful for the inspiration that hit you at 2 A.M. and that became our joint path of purpose! Thanks for having the brilliant idea to bring Rosemary on board and let her do her thing. We've only just begun and I can't wait to see what I will learn from you next!

To Dr. Rosemary Laird, my thanks for setting the bar so high! As a mom, a healing professional, a wife, an advocate, you name it; Rosemary is the best at it, all with a modest smile and a determination that doesn't accept defeat. The late night e-mails proved one more thing to me - Rosemary doesn't sleep. Ever! Thanks for pushing Jamie and me to focus our thoughts and meet our deadlines.

I will always be grateful to all of our care advocates at each of our Leeza's Place locations. This is solid, strong, loving and resourceful sisterhood. I marvel at your goodness and your caring hearts.

To Victor Starsia and Richard Day Gore, our editors at LaChance Publishing who believed in us and our idea even when we weren't sure, thanks for your faith in us and our mission. We are proud to be part of your roster of books that inspire, educate and empower. To literary agent extraordinaire Jan Miller, thanks for being the first one up to the plate with support for this project and for encouraging me to write.

Finally, thank you to each and every sleep-deprived, courageous caregiver whose life experiences became part of this book. You have hearts of gold and nerves of steel. We are proud to tell your story.

—Leeza Gibbons

■ ■ ■

My gratitude begins with Carmen and Patricia De Angelis. As extraordinary parents, and in their professional roles as teacher and nurse, I found valuable role models for leading a purposeful and balanced life. To my husband, Dr. Tim Laird, my deepest thanks for his honest critique of this book and the gift of time to write. To our children Ben, Anne, Sarah, and Katherine, thank you for being my source of constant love and encouragement.

As this book was being written, I had the privilege of being among the many dedicated individuals working to make Brevard County, Florida a community offering the highest quality health care and community resources for seniors and for caregivers of all ages. I am deeply grateful to the Health First Foundation, and in particular Larry Garrison, for their ongoing support of our Leeza's Place. That support enables our Leeza Care Advocates and the many Leeza's Place volunteers to give caregivers the support they need in their time of profound challenge. The caregivers of Health First Leeza's Place helped critique early versions of this book and their feedback was invaluable.

Heartfelt thanks to the team of associates who work alongside me at the Health First Aging Institute. Their dedication to our patients and caregivers inspires me every day. To our patients and caregivers I offer my gratitude for helping me understand your challenges and needs. I am humbled by your courage, resilience, and capacity to love in the face of life-altering change.

—Rosemary DeAngelis Laird

■ ■ ■

My mother always said, "To know oneself is to know the world." My mom, Dr. Arlene Huysman, passed away while I was writing this book, and I am proud to acknowledge her profound and inspiring influence on me. A born caregiver, psychologist and mom, she taught me through her love of life, her protective maternal energy and her tenacious passion how important it was to help myself first and then help others. She saved my life, and she is my hero and the emotional compass for my own healing journey. All my efforts at The Leeza Gibbons Memory Foundation are in honor of her power, spirit and grace. I also thank her husband, Pedro Camacho, who took care of Mom's mind, body and soul until she left this world. The years she spent well and ill were also years she knew she could find comfort and genuine love from him, her friends and fans as we all became planets orbiting around her as the Sun. I am deeply grateful for his love and devotion.

Thanks to my beautiful wife Betsy, who always supported my efforts, never questioning the countless nights spent working to bring Leeza's Place and this book to life. Her unconditional acceptance of my maniacal need to impact the world of mental health and healing was invaluable. She and the entire Bergner family were loving caregivers for my dear mother-in-law, also named Betsy, who we also lost during the writing of this book.

Thanks to my father, Michel Huysman, Esq., and his wonderful wife, Carol. There are no two people who give care to each other with greater love, adoration and selflessness. They exemplify the unique strength of a committed couple and they truly grasp the concept of "taking your oxygen first."

A deeply loving thank you to my dear and supportive sister, Pam Koretsky LCSW, who along with my mom inspired me to pursue a clinical career. She is the best geriatric clinical social worker I know. She, her husband, Steven and my talented beautiful niece Andrea have my deep gratitude.

Special thanks goes to my therapist, Dr. Dominic Callahan, whose involvement in my life has allowed me the opportunity to become aware, to transform and feel true self love every day. Finally, thanks to the "spiritual street gang" at the Leeza Gibbons Memory Foundation. This book could never have been completed without the powerful daily efforts of Bonnie Bonomo, Joyce Kennedy and

Sue Coates; Kathy Miller and Kim Jackson; Stefanie Elkins; Yael Wyte, MSW; Marissa Chapa; Maxine Vieyra; Verma Castellanos; Susan Bredau; Sean DePue; Zuen Cruz; Miguel Gutierrez and Maribel Quiala, LCSW; Jeffrey Steinberg, M.D.; Letty Sanchez and Julia Kiska.

Thanks to our "spiritual street gang" of Leeza Care Advocates, the mainstay of our Foundation. They have all taught Leeza and myself so much over the years and have helped us steer this wonderful organization in the right direction.

And finally thanks to our Leeza's Place partners around the country. Without the support of Dr. George Rapier of the WellMed Medical Group, Beth Garrow of Provena St. Joseph Medical Center, Frank Sacco of Memorial Hospital System, Paula Kupiec of Circle of Care and John Calderone of Olympia Medical Hospital, our ability to serve caregivers would be impossible.

—*James Huysman*

PART I:

KNOWLEDGE IS POWER

Once men are caught up in an event, they cease to be afraid. Only the unknown frightens men.

—Antoine de Saint-Exupéry

CHAPTER 1

Why "Take Your Oxygen First"?

"Take your oxygen first!"

All of us who have traveled by airplane have heard this phrase during the pre-flight instructions, when the flight attendants explain the use of the emergency oxygen masks. When the masks fall, it's a warning that there will be only a few seconds before every person on board will lose consciousness. If you're traveling with a young child or an elderly person, your natural reaction is to make sure he or she is safe first, before you help yourself. But if you think about it for a moment, you realize that if you ignore your own need for oxygen, there is a good chance you may be unable to help your loved one, and if that happens, you may put both yourself and your loved one in danger of serious injury or worse. The meaning of these instructions then becomes crystal clear: if you don't take care of *yourself* first, you'll be unable to care for your loved ones in their time of need.

To learn that a loved one has a progressive memory loss disorder can be as shocking as seeing that oxygen mask suddenly fall from the ceiling. It's a signal that your life is about to change; that a tremendous responsibility is about to be thrust upon you and that frightening decisions must be made. Most of all, it's a signal that you must act fast to ensure your own well being so that you'll be able to give the best care possible to your loved one in the coming years.

But how do you put your own needs ahead of your loved ones?

After all, most of us have been raised to believe that self sacrifice is a virtue. While raising our families, self sacrifice is automatic: we put the needs of our families first. In fact, in our society, self-sacrifice is expected. We're taught from a young age that we are "bad" or "self-ish" if we help ourselves before we help others. To be sure, in nearly every respect, taking responsibility for others and putting others first is a wonderful human quality, a positive attribute that nurtures our personal relationships and enhances the well being of society as a whole. But in the context of giving care to a person with a chronic illness, and in particular, to a person with a memory loss disorder, a rigid belief in the idea of self sacrifice actually *prevents* one from giving the best care one possibly can.

When you neglect your own physical, emotional and spiritual needs, you cannot possibly give effective care to a loved one. Ask yourself this: if you are not feeling well or you have neglected your own physical fitness and have no physical energy, how will you be able to keep the extra hours you'll need for all the additional work caregiving requires? If you're depressed to the point where you can't face getting out of bed, how can you keep your loved one and the rest of your family positive and moving forward? The enormous demands placed upon caregivers often result in their own serious illnesses and even in their deaths; frequently, the death of a caregiver means that no one is left to care for the person who needed care in the first place. That's why the expression "take your oxygen first" is so appropriate to the world of caregiving, particularly when caring for one with a progressive memory disorder. The oxygen mask drops with the diagnosis. If you don't take that oxygen, your life can careen out of control, ending with a disaster to your health, emotions, and spirit that reaches far beyond the individual with the diagnosis.

To make matters worse, there can be a great deal of shame and stigma attached to the idea of caregiving. Caregivers are often described as "martyrs" and "victims." To many, caregiving is often associated with *codependency*, a mental health challenge in which a person cares too much for another's struggles, often enabling bad behavior (e.g., excessive drinking) in the one being cared for. These associations cause caregivers to avoid being labeled a "caregiver" and, as a result, they fail to seek help for themselves.

Unfortunately, in our society very little is being done to educate and support caregivers and their families, perhaps because of the negative stigma associated with caregiving. It's an enormous problem. There are currently over *50 million* Americans whose well being is being seriously compromised by the burdens of caregiving. This number will grow as the baby boomer generation ages. By 2020, we expect the ranks of caregivers to expand to some 80 million. If burnout, fatigue and illness become the norm for this group, medical costs will skyrocket. The potential toll this will take not only on the individuals and their families, but on society in general, is truly monumental.

At Leeza's Place, we find this as shocking as it is unacceptable, and we want to reverse this trend. Arming yourself with knowledge and support right away can reduce the strain on your entire family by helping you understand your role and the issues you'll face. Once educated, you are less likely to become so demoralized, isolated and overwhelmed that the well being of everyone around you suffers. A strong and healthy caregiver can significantly improve the quality of life for *everyone*: the individual, the family and society.

You may be feeling overwhelmed now, but by applying the practices we use at Leeza's Place to your own life it's possible for you to become a healthier person while giving care to someone else. Leeza's Place follows what we call the "Three E's": *Education, Empowerment,* and *Energy.* Education increases your knowledge about the disease you are facing, about better ways to manage your loved one's illness and about the need to nurture your physical, emotional and spiritual well being so that you can meet the challenges of giving care to your loved one. Knowledge frees us from unnecessary and destructive anger, guilt, depression and other negative emotions so typical of caregivers and gives us the confidence we need to move forward.

Once you are Educated, you'll be able to Empower yourself through specific actions. Empowered caregivers have the strength to take responsibility for their own well-being and do something with their knowledge. Together, Education and Empowerment lead to Energy. Energy is the basis of life; it's the means by which we all can live rich and fulfilling lives no matter what is thrown at us; without it you are unable to keep up, let alone find meaning and joy every day. By making The Three E's part of your life, you can rebuild your energy and discover a richer experience for your loved ones and yourself no matter what challenges you face.

Take Your Oxygen First will show you how the three Es can be applied to your own caregiving experience. You'll join with Leeza and the Gibbons family on their journey of caregiving for Jean, and see how many of the situations they faced mirror your own—a moving example of the universal needs, challenges and potential triumphs of caregivers like you.

We'll begin by exploring the disorders suffered by our loved ones, how they are diagnosed, how they affect the mind and body, and the treatments available to fight them. We'll also give you information and advice on the best way to get the proper care for your loved one, how to navigate the health care system and how to make sure you are doing all you possibly can for your loved one.

Next, we'll show you how to take care of your body through proper exercise, good nutrition, brain fitness and getting a good night's sleep so that you can face each day with more confidence, greater strength, energy and alertness, and avoid the bad habits that can lead to illness, emotional distress and ultimately impact the life of your loved one.

We'll then turn our attention to taking care of your emotional health and show you how you can avoid the common problems of denial, guilt, anger and depression that so many caregivers face, to help you retain a vital sense of yourself even as you are assailed by the day to day rigors of caring for your loved one. You'll find out about the problems faced by Leeza and her family during the emotional roller coaster of caring for Jean and how they found ways to make the experience a positive one.

Finally, we'll help you learn how to find meaning in your life as a caregiver; the great comfort and joy that can be found in caring for a loved one with a memory loss disorder. We'll face with you the many challenges to the family that a memory loss disorder can bring, and show you how to bridge the generations of your family with creative and interesting activities that can enrich your life and the lives of those around you.

Throughout, you'll find useful tips from Leeza's dad, Carlos, Sr., called "Carlos, Sr.'s O2 for Caregivers", which he learned while taking care of Jean.

Ultimately, you'll learn how caregiving for someone with a memory disorder—potentially one of the most physically, emotionally and spiritually catastrophic experiences anyone will ever know—can actually turn you into a stronger and more capable person, with a clear sense of meaning and purpose in life. By the time you finish this book, we hope you'll see that when you care for yourself first, you ensure that your loved one gets the best possible care you can give.

So go ahead, take your oxygen first! You need it. And what's more: *you deserve it.*

CHAPTER 2

Understanding Memory Loss Disorders

Leeza: Mom first began showing symptoms of the disease when she was in her late 50's. Mom was in charge of paying the household bills every month, and she always kept a calendar of which bills needed to be paid when. I remember Dad telling us Mom had confessed to him one day that she had paid the same bill three times. So, in a way, it was really Mom who forced the family to begin to think that something was wrong.

After that, we all started noticing things about her behavior that just "weren't Mom." She began repeating things she had just said over and over. Then her personality began to change. Mom, who had never cursed a day in her life, started using profanity. She began raging and screaming at Dad with paranoid and outlandish accusations, saying he had never loved her and that he was trying to kill her. You can imagine how crushing these words were to hear. She would say the most horrible, hurtful things to Cammy, just out of the blue. They just destroyed my kid sister. I remember one Easter, when the family put together an egg hunt for the kids at my home. Mom, who lived for her grandchildren, just stood in the yard, pulling on her lower lip, ignoring the kids and seemingly in another world. Another time, I took her out to lunch at a local café. While I was paying the bill, Mom walked out to the front of the restaurant. I found her sitting in the back seat of someone else's car. But one of the most frightening things I remember from those days was the fearful look in her eyes she sometimes got, like she didn't know where she was or who the people around her were.

Still, we weren't able to bring ourselves to believe that Mom had the same disease that had taken her mother. We all thought that Mom, who was quite a social drinker, may have crossed over the line into alcoholism. I recall being on the phone with the family one night, talking about Mom's behavior and what to do about it, when she picked up the extension and said, "Leeza Kim, I know what you're doing. I know you're going to send me to that Henry Ford place." We were talking about sending her to the Betty Ford Center for alcoholism.

The really sad part of the whole situation was that we waited so long before we finally took her to the doctor and got a diagnosis, which didn't happen until she was 63. I guess it was a combination of Dad covering up for her behavior whenever one of the kids raised the issue, our not really understanding what was happening to her, and I guess not wanting to believe that our wonderful mother might have such a terrible illness. But knowing what I know now, if I had to do it all over again, I would have taken her to the doctor at the first sign of trouble.

As the Gibbons family and countless other families experienced, the diagnosis of a degenerative memory disorder is a life-changing event, for the person diagnosed as well as for that person's spouse, family and friends. It creates a whirlwind of emotion: an acute sense of loss, grief for the afflicted loved one, anger about one's lack of control over the disease. But a diagnosis can also bring a sense of relief, the relief of knowing the cause of the problem. Understanding the disease means we can act, rather than flail about in the dark. Knowledge enables the caregiver to adjust more easily to the changes the illness will bring, allows all concerned to better prepare for the future and can help improve the present and future quality of the lives of everyone involved. Learning what the disease looks like, what to expect, and what steps to take can also help our loved ones manage their own experience with less anxiety and allows them to take a more active role in their own care.

> *Leeza: I always love it when Oprah says, "When you know better, you do better." I think that's especially true of caregivers. That's why we encourage people to get educated early and get a diagnosis as soon as possible. Rather than creating more hopelessness, knowing what the condition is allows you precious time to hear your loved ones' wants, needs and desires and allows them to participate in their own care. It also prevents a lack of knowledge from creating situations that we might later regret. For example, many people tell me they wish they'd known their mother had Alzheimer's earlier because they would have spent far less time correcting her and trying to convince her to do things differently. Alzheimer's patients cannot join us in our world. We must join them in theirs.*

In this chapter you'll learn about how we think, how memories are made and about the disorders that cause memory loss. In particular, you'll learn about the most common cause of memory loss, Alzheimer's disease, how it affects those who have it and how to best manage its effects. Caring for someone with a degenerative health condition presents intense demands and challenges. Learning how to meet these challenges is a process; it doesn't happen right away. But understanding more about the disease can help you better take the caregiving challenges in stride. Remember, knowledge is power!

The Brain

The human brain is a four pound collection of nerve cells with three main components: the *cerebrum*, the *cerebellum*, and the *brain stem*. The brain communicates with the rest of the body through the brain stem's connection to the spinal cord and its collection of nerves that extend to all parts of the body, all of which together are known as the *nervous system*. Through these connections, the brain controls all of our activities, including our intellectual processes, our emotions, our physical actions, and our behaviors.

These activities are controlled by different sections of the brain. The *cerebrum* consists of the *cerebral cortex* (grey matter), where thinking processes reside, and white matter, which helps transmit nerve impulses between brain sections. The cerebrum is divided into lobes which each have a specific set of functions. The *frontal lobe*, located in the front of the brain, is associated with personality, problem solving, abstract thought, and skilled movement. The *parietal lobes*, located just above and behind the frontal lobe, receive sensory input such as pain, taste and touch. They are also responsible for *visuospatial* abilities, such as understanding the distance between oneself and another object. The *temporal lobes*, along the sides the brain, are involved with hearing and language comprehension, perception and parts of the process of memory. The *occipital lobe*, located at the back of the brain, is responsible for vision. Certain internal sections of the cerebrum also provide special functions. For example, the processes involved with making and retrieving memories are managed in an area called the *hippocampus*.

MAJOR SECTIONS OF THE BRAIN

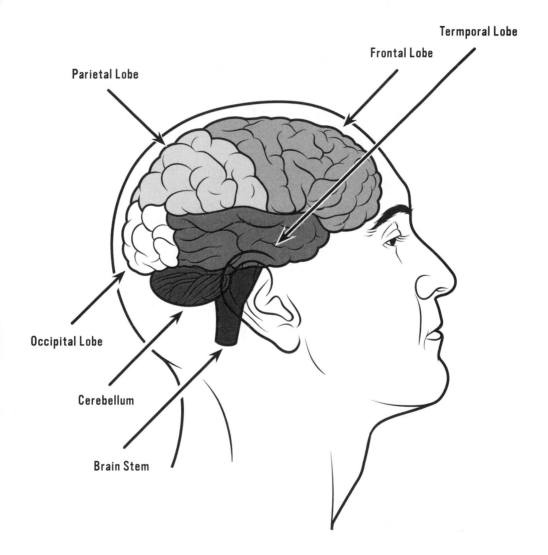

Termporal Lobe

Frontal Lobe

Parietal Lobe

Occipital Lobe

Cerebellum

Brain Stem

How We Think

Thinking is a complex set of *cognitive processes* performed by the brain that include perception, attention, memory, judgment, and reasoning. The word "cognitive" comes from a Latin term meaning "to know" and these processes are the way we learn and how we apply what we learn to make decisions, create, remember and communicate. The basic working unit of thinking in the brain, and in the entire nervous system throughout the body, is the *neuron*. Neurons are structures that allow different parts of the brain to communicate with each other by *electrical impulses*, which are the means by which we think and then act.

An electrical impulse is created when a neuron is stimulated by something like hearing a friend's voice on the phone or by stubbing one's toe. These stimuli cause an electrical impulse to be sent across the neuron to its tip, where chemicals called *neurotransmitters* are released. These chemicals pass to the next neuron and stimulate it, which in turn stimulates the next neuron, and the next and the next, until the impulse reaches its destination, which may be the part of the brain that houses the memory of the friend's voice or the muscles that allow you to rub your toe.

How Memories Are Made

Memories are made and stored using many different parts of the cerebrum. Let's say you meet someone named Isabelle. As you are greeting her, the image of her face is registering in the occipital lobe of the brain as a *visual sensory perception*. Then Isabelle tells you her name, and that *aural sensory perception* (hearing the name Isabelle) is registered in the temporal lobe of your brain. Both of these items are now "stored" as part of what is known as *short-term memory*.

If you then leave Isabelle's presence and never hear of or encounter her again, it's unlikely that you will retain a long-term memory of her face or her name. Only information that is encoded or consolidated through attention, repetition or associated ideas results in the creation of a new long-term memory. For example, if Isabelle hands you a business card and you see her name written on it, or in conversation you find out you both enjoy the same restaurant, it's more likely this information will help consolidate her name and face as a *long-term memory*. It is the hippocampus that will coordinate and encode all of the bits of information you stored about Isabelle's name and face so that you can recognize her at a later date.

As we get older, all parts of the body change. Some changes are easy to see, like grey hair and wrinkles. Other changes are less obvious. In the brain, the number of nerve cells (neurons) decreases and some thought processes become less efficient. Memory is one of those areas that slow down some for just about everyone. For example, it can take longer to remember the name of your friend on the church committee. This mild form of memory loss comes naturally with aging and does not negatively impact one's ability to function. But this is *not* the same type of memory loss and disrupted thinking that come with memory loss disorders.

What Is Degenerative Memory Loss?

Degenerative memory loss disorders cause *dementia* and dramatically impact how a person functions and the quality of his life. Dementia is best understood as a progressive loss of brain function that affects memory, communication, learning and behavior. Of all the memory loss disorders, Alzheimer's disease is the most common form, accounting for about fifty to sixty-five percent of all dementia cases. We will look at Alzheimer's disease in detail later in this chapter. But other disorders are also responsible for degenerative memory loss. They include the following:

VASCULAR DEMENTIA

Vascular dementia is caused by one or more *strokes* occurring in specific areas of the brain. Stroke is an umbrella term that refers to any interruption of blood flow to the brain. In some cases, Alzheimer's disease and vascular dementia can occur together. One difference between the two disorders is that memory loss is one of the first symptoms of Alzheimer's, while with vascular dementia, memory problems can occur later in the disease process. More often, the first symptoms of vascular dementia include difficulty with language, speech, and vision, with memory loss arising later.

Rarely occurring before the age of 65, vascular dementia is not truly "progressive" like Alzheimer's disease. Instead, the condition worsens in surges as large numbers of brain cells are suddenly deprived of their blood supply as a result of multiple strokes. You might think of it as a "staircase" progression, worsening in fits and starts rather than by a slow, continuous acceleration of disease. There's no cure for vascular dementia, but some relief is possible through medications and lifestyle changes.

LEWY BODY DISEASE

Lewy body disease, sometimes referred to as *dementia with Lewy bodies* or *dementia associated with Parkinson's disease* is another very common cause of dementia, accounting for approximately 15% to 20% of cases that start after the age of 65. The name for the disease comes from the presence in the brain of abnormal round deposits, called Lewy bodies, which contain damaged nerve cells. Lewy body disease has symptoms similar to both Alzheimer's and Parkinson's disease, and it is often present in those with Parkinson's disease. In fact, about 35% of Parkinson's disease patients develop *Parkinson's disease dementia*, which is a Lewy body dementia. Lewy body disease affects memory, language, the ability to judge distances and the ability to complete simple actions. People with this form of dementia suffer hallucinations and they may also experience falls because their abilities to judge distances and coordinate physical movement are disrupted. The cause of Lewy body disease is unknown. There is no cure, although there is hope that drugs now in development will be able to delay the onset of symptoms, which often progress much more rapidly than those of Alzheimer's disease.

FRONTOTEMPORAL LOBAR DEMENTIA

Frontotemporal lobar dementia (FTLD), which includes *Picks disease*, refers to a group of dementias caused by the loss of brain tissue in the frontal and temporal areas of the brain. In their advanced stages, the symptoms of FTLD and Alzheimer's disease often appear very similar, but they differ dramatically early on, and the FTLD disorders can occur earlier and progress faster than Alzheimer's disease. Signs and symptoms may include inappropriate sexual behavior, the loss of concern over personal appearance and hygiene, apathy and a lack of concern for others, speech and language difficulties and memory loss in their later stages. There is no treatment to slow the progression of FTLD, although anti-depressant and psychiatric medications have been shown to improve some symptoms and, while they have not been evaluated for this use, the medications used to treat Alzheimer's disease are often prescribed for FTLD patients.

CREUTZFELDT - JAKOB DISEASE

Creutzfeldt-Jakob disease (CJD) is a rare, degenerative brain disorder caused by a misshapen form of a protein found in the brain called a *prion*. Some forms of CJD are related to the highly publicized "mad cow disease", but most are due to spontaneous genetic mutations. In the early stages of the disease, patients may have failing memory, behavioral changes, a lack of physical coordination and visual disturbances. As the illness progresses, mental deterioration becomes pronounced and involuntary movements, blindness, weakness of the arms and legs, and coma may occur. The current treatment for CJD aims to alleviate the symptoms and make the patient as comfortable as possible. This disease progresses quickly, and is usually fatal within a year of diagnosis.

ALZHEIMER'S DISEASE

According to the Alzheimer's Association, one in every ten families in this country has a relative suffering from Alzheimer's disease. Of the four million people with Alzheimer's disease in the United States, 70% live at home, often receiving part or full-time care from family members. Alarmingly, due to the longer life spans now being enjoyed by so many, it is expected that the population of Alzheimer's disease patients will double every 20 years.[1]

But the disease it is not limited to the aged population. Alzheimer's is sometimes diagnosed in people in their thirties or forties. The Alzheimer's Association estimates that there are between 220,000 and 640,000 Americans with *early onset* Alzheimer's disease (that which is

---

1 *Alzheimer's disease: Unraveling the Mystery.* United States Department of Health and Human Services, National Institute on Aging; 1995. N.I.H. publication 95-3782.

diagnosed in persons who are under the age of 60) and other dementias. Because it is the most common of all the memory loss disorders, we'll take a closer look at the causes of Alzheimer's disease, the potential symptoms and duration of the disease, and the different challenges caregivers may face in each phase of its progression.

In 1906 Dr. Alois Alzheimer, a German physician, noticed changes in the brain tissue of a woman who had died of an unusual mental illness. He found within the brain abnormal clumps, now called *amyloid plaques,* and tangled bundles of fibers within the patient's neurons, now called *neurofibrillary tangles.* Today, these plaques and tangles are considered to be the hallmarks of the presence of Alzheimer's disease, although scientists have yet to determine the exact role they play in the disorder. It is clear, however, that a person with Alzheimer's disease progressively loses healthy brain tissue, which causes a steady decline in mental abilities. In fact, by the time Alzheimer's is diagnosed, nerve cells that process, store, and retrieve information have been degenerating and dying for some time. This degeneration eventually destroys a person's memory and his ability to learn, reason, make judgments, communicate, and carry out routine daily activities.

Diagnosing Alzheimer's Disease

Diagnosing Alzheimer's disease requires an evaluation by a physician with experience in looking for the characteristic patterns of the disease. The physician will ask the patient and his family for a detailed history of the changes in intellect, emotion, and behavior they have noticed, and will perform cognitive testing, brain imaging, and special blood tests. Physicians trained in geriatrics and neurology are usually the most experienced in diagnosing the disease. In many cases, primary care physicians with backgrounds in internal and family medicine are also well prepared to identify and diagnose dementias. Unfortunately, most diagnoses of Alzheimer's disease are delayed until more than two years after the first symptoms appear. A lack of awareness on the part of families and medical personnel, denial of symptoms and the stigma surrounding the disease may all play a role in delaying diagnosis. This delay can have a serious medical impact on those affected, since medications to slow the illness' progress are most effective in its early stages. An early diagnosis also enables caregivers to respond to its symptoms more effectively by, for example, changing the home environment, which can significantly improve the quality of life for the loved one. Caregivers are also likely to have more patience with loved ones if they are aware of and understand the disease early on. Having an early diagnosis also means that a loved one and his caregiver can talk together about the future, making decisions together before the ability of the loved one to participate is lost.

Is Alzheimer's Disease Inherited?

It is generally believed that a combination of genetic predisposition and physical changes in the brain lead to Alzheimer's disease and the other dementing illnesses. There is a strong genetic link between early onset Alzheimer's disease and the presence of a gene expressing a mutation known as *trisomy 21* that is responsible for Down's syndrome, a disorder that causes developmental delays during childhood. There are some rare families with known genetic defects that lead to several family members being afflicted, often with early onset illness.

In most cases of Alzheimer's disease, the genetic risk is not as clear. Only 5% to 10% of Alzheimer's disease cases occur in people who have at least two first-degree relatives (a parent, brother, sister or children) with a history of Alzheimer's disease. The most evaluated risk factor is the gene known as *apoE*. Inheritance of a version of this gene is regarded as a risk factor in nearly 50% of all cases of late-onset Alzheimer's disease. But the presence of the apoE gene is not the complete answer. Genetics experts agree that there are other, as yet unidentified, genes that influence the development of Alzheimer's disease. Because of this uncertainty, there is no genetic test available to assess risk.

Leeza: The good thing about getting a diagnosis, at least for our family, was being able to confront the enemy and face it head-on. It was a great relief for Mom and her friends to know why she had changed.

I certainly don't live my life in fear and yet I am not naïve about my increased risk for Alzheimer's disease. I do everything I can to manage my risk and become educated about the possibility of preventing the disease, including taking vitamin supplements, following a healthy diet, exercising regularly and managing everyday stress. Memory screenings seem, in my opinion, to be a great tool in the arsenal against memory robbing illnesses. It is only when we have knowledge that we can become empowered to effect change. I have taken the memory screening tests we have on our Leeza's Place website. While it is not a tool of diagnosis, it helped me in the same way it has helped a lot of others: I breathed a sigh of relief when it showed my memory to be within a normal range. Being in the dark about something as insidious as Alzheimer's disease accomplishes nothing.

The Symptoms Of Alzheimer's Disease

Amnesic mild cognitive impairment (amnesic MCI) is a term used to identify those individuals who suffer mild memory impairment but whose other abilities and functions remain intact. Of those who are diagnosed with amnesic MCI, almost all will eventually progress to full Alzheimer's disease. Detailed testing can reveal mild memory difficulties up to eight years before a person's symptoms meet the criteria of a diagnosis of Alzheimer's disease. The time of its conversion to Alzheimer's disease and its rate of progression varies widely among individuals.

Alzheimer's disease may last from a couple of years to several decades. The average duration of the disease is between eight and twenty years. Individuals may experience a fast progression of symptoms or remain with the same symptoms for a long time. Those with early onset Alzheimer's disease tend to reach the final stage sooner, generally in three to five years. Later onset Alzheimer's disease tends to progress over a period of ten years or more. While there is a wide variation in the rate of its progression among individuals, there are common changes seen in all patients over time. Regardless of the rate of progression, the disease inevitably evolves from minor to severe.

The course of Alzheimer's disease is typically divided into three stages, with a different pattern of cognitive and physical impairment occurring at each stage. In the lists below, the changes commonly seen at the *early, middle, and late* stages are described as they typically emerge over time. However, the progression of Alzheimer's disease is far more complex and unique in its expression in particular individuals than such a breakdown can represent, and symptoms may occur earlier or later than is described, depending on the individual. What is certain is that the disease progresses first by affecting the intellectual processes, then to affecting physical activities, and finally to severely impeding the major bodily functions.

Early Stage Symptoms

Taylor (age 20): J.G. would ask me over and over and over if my boyfriend was a new boyfriend. I thought, should I remind her, or could that possibly make her feel like she's bad or even make her feel like she shouldn't try to talk to me and be involved with my life?

In general, during the early stages of Alzheimer's disease, a person may have difficulty on the job or trouble doing things the way he used to, but will often still be healthy, high functioning, and able to communicate feelings and concerns. People with mild dementia usually still function independently. Sometimes they are aware of

WHAT ARE THE WARNING SIGNS OF ALZHEIMER'S DISEASE? THE ALZHEIMER'S ASSOCIATION'S TOP 10 ARE:

- Memory loss
- Difficulty performing familiar tasks
- Problems with language
- Disorientation to time and place
- Poor or decreased judgment
- Problems with abstract thinking
- Misplacing things
- Changes in mood or behavior
- Changes in personality
- Loss of initiative

their symptoms and adapt to the changes they sense. Some, however, are not aware of their symptoms, and it is family or friends who first begin to sense something is wrong. The symptoms at this stage vary greatly from person to person, but commonly include:

Memory loss. Short term memory loss is often the first symptom experienced. The person affected may constantly lose things, or arrive at the grocery store and realize that he left his list at home, again. He might lose track of stories or conversations. Memories from long-ago are intact, but recent events may blur together. He may begin to ask repetitive questions, and to have trouble organizing his thoughts.

Aphasia. Early in the disease, a person with Alzheimer's disease starts forgetting words, especially nouns ("house," "car," "book"), and is often unable to communicate his thoughts easily. He may stop talking to avoid making mistakes.

Loss of Judgment and Ability to Make Decisions. The person affected usually finds it increasingly difficult to solve everyday problems or to respond appropriately in different situations. There is greater difficulty in doing things that require planning or making decisions, such as preparing dinner or getting the laundry done in the right order. He may suddenly be unable to balance the checkbook or pay bills on time, forget to pay or pay too much or too little. Driving can become increasingly dangerous, as he may over or under-react to situations on the road. He may forget to eat, or eat constantly. He may begin to hide things in odd places and then forget where they are hidden, or he may hide things of little or no value.

Mood and Behavioral Changes. Changes in mood can be the first sign that something is wrong. A person with early-stage Alzheimer's disease might exhibit moodiness and become withdrawn and subdued, especially in social situations, which may be due, in part, to anxiety about the uncontrollable changes in his memory. He may

CAREGIVING DURING THE EARLY STAGE OF ALZHEIMER'S DISEASE

This can be a tricky stage for families. The caregiving role is new, and you are suddenly required to help someone who may be resentful or still operates with a high degree of awareness and is reluctant to give up any independence. He lives with the memories of who he was, not as he is with degenerating cognitive abilities. It is important to step carefully and respectfully into his private space so as not to demean him or treat him as one would a child. Relationships will also need to be repaired, if they have soured, or renewed if it's been a while since you've connected well. This can actually be a time for finding your way to a deeper connection –but it will probably take work and, above all, a willingness to do it.

During this initial stage of the disease, caregivers can promote the patient's sense of well being by providing emotional support and by helping to maintain familiar activities and social contacts. It's best to focus more on what people can still do, rather than on their limitations. People in the early stages of the disease can take advantage of recreational, social, educational, and vocational programs. It's also important to begin to differentiate between the disease and the loved one: recognizing that the disease, not the loved one, is responsible for some difficult behaviors.

also be slower to respond, less energetic, and may say things or act in ways that are inappropriate. Sleep disturbances or frequent restlessness are also common.

Middle Stage Symptoms

Serious gaps in functioning are seen once the disease progresses to its middle stage. Caregivers must hone their communication skills to meet the new challenges in cognition that arise, and make the necessary changes to the home environment to meet the safety and physical needs of those affected. People in this stage become an increasing danger to themselves and are not able to maintain daily activities, such as personal hygiene and eating regularly. Symptoms associated with this phase of the disease are:

An inability to perform common tasks. Often a person with middle-stage Alzheimer's disease struggles to perform simple, routine tasks that require sequential steps, such as brushing one's teeth or showering. He will not be able to follow directions as well; even asking him to turn off a running faucet could prove futile. Using keys becomes troublesome and driving safely is no longer possible.

Increased Confusion. At this stage confusion is more common and more disruptive than in the early stage. The person loses awareness of time and the date, finds himself lost in what used to be familiar surroundings, and cannot remember people and places he once knew. He may not recognize himself or his close family. It's not uncommon for a loved one with Alzheimer's disease to wander away from home. Information will simply not be processed adequately, thus, for example, images, such as reflections in a mirror, may become impossible for him to understand.

Impaired Motor Skills. As the brain continues to lose cells, motor functioning will begin to decrease. Walking, sitting, or stand-

CAREGIVING DURING MIDDLE-STAGE ALZHEIMER'S DISEASE

This stage really brings home the reality of the disease and your role as the caregiver. It can be the most stressful time for a family. You begin to take charge of your loved one entirely as his functioning diminishes. You will have to learn to meet the ever-greater demand for intervention and care.

The challenge of finding a comfortable balance between your loved one's independence and his increased need for assistance calls for flexibility on your part. It can be a challenge to step in more often, especially when a loved one is used to being dominant. But caring at this stage demands more than a watchful eye, and your role will change from supervisor to actively taking charge of his well-being. The key is learning how to do this creatively, without engaging in power struggles or causing greater anxiety for your loved one.

By now, most Alzheimer's disease patients are living in a world that is largely unreal, but they are still connected to all their senses. Communication can be difficult, if not impossible, but you can learn to reach them and help them experience pleasurable moments in new ways. Communicating love and kindness doesn't really require words. Your loved one will respond more to your tone and body language than the actual content. One of the best ways to interact with a loved one in the middle stage of Alzheimer's disease is to engage their senses. Activities that stimulate positive sensations, such as a massage or a walk through sweet smelling gardens, are enjoyable at any stage.

ing without help can all become difficult as balance and awareness of the surroundings diminish. Often, the loved one will need help understanding how to use the toilet. Self-feeding will probably require extra measures, such as using only a spoon and cutting food up before it is served.

Personality changes. Some of the more difficult symptoms of middle-stage Alzheimer's disease are the personality changes, which are more dramatic now and less connected to reality. You might notice sudden mood swings, distrust in others, increased stubbornness or social withdrawal. Depression, restlessness, anxiety or aggression are common, and inappropriate behaviors such as unfounded accusations, threats, cursing, kicking, hitting or biting may occur. He may begin to experience delusions and hallucinations, such as believing that people are out to trick or attack him, or he may see, hear, smell or taste things that are not there. Now is also the time you might begin to notice compulsive, repetitive behaviors such as hand wringing, tissue shredding or inappropriate sexual behavior, such as mistaking another individual for a spouse or disrobing or masturbating in public.

Leeza: Daddy was unbelievably understanding with Mom and I have such respect for how he managed it all. They would go out in public, and Mom would, as many people do in this stage of the disease, behave inappropriately. She would often eat off plates belonging to others, but still Daddy would take her out. Even when she had her bra on the outside of her blouse, he would say, "You look beautiful Honey, let's go." Sometimes Dad would discretely pass out a card to the people working at the restaurant that read, "Please be patient, my partner tonight is dealing with memory issues." He didn't want to embarrass her by talking about her to others as though she were an object. They were a familiar sight at their local haunts and she would often tell people herself that she had the disease. I remember one time when we were all at a fund-raiser and we couldn't find my mother. We panicked. I eventually spotted her in a corner of the ballroom where everyone was dressed in formal attire. She was ripping off her turquoise sequined gown. It was horrifying. Dad came over and tried to make it O.K. while none of us spoke our fears out loud. But we knew her disease had claimed another part of her soul.

Late-Stage Symptoms

Lexi (age 19): As humans we have the ability to connect memory with faces, places, smells, sights, emotions and touch. It is the essence of who we are. It's all so rich and full; it's everything. I could never imagine losing all of the memories I have built. What happens when they evaporate? The disease that took my grandmother was devil-sent. It steals people's dreams and memories and replaces them with a state of nothingness. At least that is the fear. The people affected experience on of the things that we as humans have never been able to grasp and the thing of which we are most afraid: nothingness.

During the last stage of Alzheimer's disease, caregivers struggle to find a hint of the person they once knew. The emotional instability and delusions of the middle stage are replaced by serious physical problems requiring care twenty-four hour a day, seven days a week. A loved one with late-stage Alzheimer's disease loses his ability to respond to his environment. In the end, the diseased brain can no longer support bodily functions. If the person does not die of other

CAREGIVING DURING THE LATE STAGE OF ALZHEIMER'S DISEASE

Many caregivers feel some relief to have made it through the difficulties of the middle stage of the disease. The battles and emotional upheavals have settled down and because your loved one is now bedridden (or chair bound) there is less fear that he will hurt himself or those around him. It's easier to take charge now that your loved one is no longer struggling for autonomy in any way; your job is clearer and simpler in this respect.

Because people with late stage Alzheimer's disease are unable to make decisions about their own medical care, it is important to consider these issues long before they arise. At some point in the later stages of the disease it may become important to get hospice care, or place your loved one where he can receive the extensive care he now needs. But there are still ways you can care for your loved one, even at this late stage. He won't recognize you or be able to communicate verbally, but you can still show him reassurance and love. You might spend time brushing his hair or rub his hands with lotion. You could read out loud, soothing him with the rhythmic sound of your voice, or play a video with colorful images to interest him. Ultimately, you want to help your loved one live out his life with as much comfort, respect, and dignity as possible.

causes, Alzheimer's disease eventually causes death. The symptoms at this stage include:

Loss of Motor Control. The most dramatic symptom of this stage is the inability to sit, stand, or walk. Smiling, swallowing, and holding the head up becomes increasingly impossible. Joints may also be stiffer and unable to bend without assistance. Most people are bedridden or chair-bound by this stage.

Loss of Appetite. Interest in food decreases dramatically, perhaps because of the amount of effort required to chew and swallow. He may choke, forget to swallow, or refuse to eat.

Physical Problems. The skin becomes more and more prone to bruises and pressure ulcers (often called bed sores). It is common to see weight loss and a loss of control of the bowels and bladder.

Loss of Speech. Where your loved one only struggled for the right word before, now he may be unable to make words or even sounds. The facial muscles, like the rest of the body, are functioning less and less and they may appear to be "frozen" much of the time.

Compromised Immune System. Because of the general deterioration of the body, the immune system no longer protects your loved one as it used to. He is at high risk for contracting infections, and even a mild cold can turn into a serious problem.

TREATMENT FOR ALZHEIMER'S DISEASE

It is often said there is no "treatment" for Alzheimer's disease. While it is true that the disease is incurable, there is a distinction between a condition that is incurable and one that is untreatable. There are drug therapies to treat some of the symptoms of Alzheimer's disease, to stabilize the loss of thought processes and to decrease the troubling symptoms of depression or aggression experienced by many and which can improve the overall quality of life of the patient as well as the caregiver. The decision to use these drugs should be made through discussions among the patient, the caregivers and the patient's physician.

There are two classes of drugs available today for the treatment of the disease. *Acetylcholinesterase inhibitors* are drugs that increase the level of *acetylcholine* in the brain, one of the neurotransmitter chemicals necessary for cognitive function. These include Aricept (donepezil), Exelon (rivastigmine) and Razadyne (galantamine). In patients with mild to moderate Alzheimer's disease, these drugs are able to slow the loss of cognitive abilities for as long as eighteen months and can improve certain functional abilities, emotional symptoms, and common complications such as hallucinations. Their side effects are relatively few and can include digestive discomfort and sleep changes.

Namenda (memantine) works by blocking another neurotransmitter, called *glutamate,* from affecting a nerve receptor known as NMDA. While glutamate is important for the development of long term memories, it is believed that too much may be harmful to nerve receptors and may contribute to the development of Alzheimer's disease. As with the first class of drugs, this drug has minimal side effects that include headache, dizziness, constipation, and euphoria. Both classes of drugs were originally approved for those with middle to late stage Alzheimer's disease but are now often prescribed for patients in its early stages as well.

In addition to the treatment of cognitive changes, there is often a need to treat the emotional or behavioral symptoms of the disease. The most common emotional symptom associated with Alzheimer's disease is a depressed mood together with irritability or agitation. If you are faced with this, first seek out non-drug strategies that might help you manage your loved one's symptoms, such as counseling or increasing daytime activities by, for example, attending an adult day program. In other cases medications are a necessary part of the treatment. *Selective serotonin reuptake inhibitors* (SSRIs) are a class of antidepressants used in the treatment of these symptoms and which are relatively free of side effects. More serious behaviors, such as physical aggression, may require other behavior modification strategies and/or drug treatments. However, medications to control these behaviors have more serious side effects, including the worsening of cognitive abilities and difficulty walking, which could lead to an increased incidence of falls. It is best to avoid using these strong drugs unless it becomes absolutely necessary. Your physician can help guide you in the treatment of these symptoms.

Education - The Payoff

"It took a long time for us to face our fears and get a diagnosis for Jean," Carlos, Sr. recalls. "But we were glad we did, even though it was devastating. Just knowing what we were up against gave us a starting point. Eventually, we understood that we were powerless to save Jean, but at least we could go through the process with less confusion and fear."

If you've developed a good, basic grasp of the science of the disorder afflicting your loved one, you've taken one of the biggest steps you can towards making your own life more stress-free. You're less intimidated by health plans, prescriptions and doctor's visits. You have a better idea of what's "behind" your loved one's sometimes baffling behavior. You're well on your way to making the first of the Three E's, Education, a "feather in your cap." And you have a head start on the next E, Empowerment. You now have a base of knowledge which will empower you when dealing with doctors and other medical professionals. You need to know how and where to get help, how to find the right doctors and work with them to take the best care of your loved one—which ultimately will help you get through your caregiving days with a new sense of energy and peace.

CHAPTER 3

Finding Help

*L*eeza: *Without Mom's insistence, we probably wouldn't have had a diagnosis for a couple of years. What happens in the rhythm of relationships is that spouses cover for each other and it becomes a dance so well performed that those outside the circle can't notice the nuances of changes that are happening. As a long distance caregiver, I had no idea how rapidly Mom was declining. Mom and Dad didn't want to rock the boat with their doctor, and Mom had been fairly healthy, so the doctor wasn't seeing any radical changes in her. On the days of the doctor visits she was sometimes asymptomatic. That's a tough place for caregivers. Even though there will be those days where your loved one will be very present and lucid, don't be fooled by that. Be grateful for it, but listen to your intuition. Continue to impress upon your doctor what you suspect. I encourage people to challenge their doctors, to write out their questions before the appointment and to never go alone to the appointments. If you think there is something wrong, chances are you're right.*

Once they had Jean's diagnosis, Leeza and her family quickly found that doctors and medical appointments became a regular part of their lives. And like them, you will need to become proactive in your search for medical care for your loved one, because successful caregiving begins with the right doctor. You need a doctor who listens to your loved one's values and wishes, and who bases his or her medical advice on that critical foundation. But how do you find doctors who listen and who can help raise your comfort and confidence?

Barbara, one of our guests at Leeza's Place, was alarmed when her mother was diagnosed with the flu. Fearing that she might be contagious, her mother didn't want Barbara to visit her. But they kept in touch by phone until Barbara began to feel that her mother was not recovering as quickly as she should. Disregarding her mother's protests, Barbara went to her and found her in very poor condition, not taking her medications and not eating properly. Soon afterwards Barbara's mother was hospitalized to and spent weeks in the intensive care unit. Today she is back home and living independently once again, but now with weekly, and sometimes more frequent, visits from her children.

Months later, Barbara told us of her fears during the ordeal: "What worried me the most was being the one responsible for making sure Mother got all the care possible; I wanted to make sure I learned what I needed to know. If she was going to die, even after everything that *could* be done for her *had* been done, then it was out of my hands. But the healthcare professionals involved in her care were focused exclusively on the lifesaving part of the work, which left me on my own. So instead of being able to rely on the medical professionals caring for mother, I had to rely on my friends and colleagues for advice on what to do."

The source of Barbara's fear was that she could not be sure if she was doing all she could for her mother. She worried that she wasn't asking the right questions, finding the right doctors, keeping her mother away from medical errors and making the right decisions. Medical professionals often believe that the caregiver is looking for "the cure" when, just as often, the caregiver understands that there is only so much that medicine can do. More important to the caregiver is the assurance that all has been done to give their loved one the best care and, if possible, additional days, months, or years of what their loved one would consider a quality life. But as caregivers and patients become immersed in the complicated and chaotic world of a hospital or health system, such clarity can be elusive at best.

The health care system's endemic lack of support for caregivers can increase the stress of an already difficult situation. But it is possible to reduce the uncertainties that lead to emotional turmoil. You can prepare for and manage a loved one's health crisis by taking the following steps and by creating a partnership of care with the doctors and the other healthcare professionals who are part of what might seem like an impenetrable health care system.

Step 1: Get Close to Your Loved One

Leeza: We knew that taking care of Mom was going to be costly and that we wanted her to have the best possible care, so as we were still sorting out our feelings of grief and anger, sadness and loss, I pushed us to move forward and look at Mom and Dad's financial situation. This is the area in which we all became a little stressed. Daddy didn't want us to worry so when we asked him, "Do you have enough insurance, do you have long term care insurance?" Daddy would say, "We're fine honey, you don't have to worry". Even so, I insisted that I come home and that we gather together just to lay everything out. When we dug into the records and financials, we found a mess. Mom was the one who kept all the files, paid all the bills and ran the "business" of their marriage. Dad wasn't able to put his hands on the information right away. When we did sort things out, we found that he didn't have adequate insurance and money was tight. Maybe it was his pride, his paternal protection or just one of the places we hide when we're hurting, but it is imperative for families to get real with each other on this issue. One of the first steps is to get a financial overview to come up with some ideas of what you may need and to begin to put together a plan.

We also knew that Dad was going to need some help taking care of Mom at home, so I came home to help him interview potential caregivers. I researched three companies and arranged for them to send over candidates. I tried to ask them all the same questions so I could compare their responses. Of course, I had already made sure that they were bonded professionals with clear backgrounds. It became a question of who Mom felt most comfortable with. It was important for us to make sure Mom knew that she was involved in the hiring process. Mom and Dad and I met with each of the candidates in the living room. The ones that didn't speak to Mom directly or spoke about her as if she wasn't in the room I immediately dismissed. When you entrust someone with this most intimate role, it's important that the family and your loved one feel comfortable. It may not be the right match the first time, but it's worth pursuing. Mom got very close to one of her caregivers and they became buddies. She gave Mom a feeling of independence. They went to exercise class; they went to get Mom's hair done. It gave Daddy a break and those were really good times for the family.

To caregivers, nothing is more comforting than knowing they are carrying out their loved one's wishes when making life-altering decisions. Don't wait for a crisis to learn your loved one's desires. First, know your loved one's wishes in the event that critical healthcare decisions need to be made on his or her behalf. Second, know what insurance and other financial resources are available to support those wishes. Include all of your important family members in these discussions, and determine well ahead of time who among you will be responsible for making these decisions and how an acute health crisis will be handled. You will then be well prepared to help when a crisis comes.

Given the complexity and fast pace of the health care system, it is best for anyone admitted to a hospital due to a health crisis such as a stroke, hip fracture or serious illness to have someone with them from the time of admission and, afterwards, for as many hours a day as possible during his or her stay. If you or another close family member cannot personally get there, enlist the help of a neighbor, friend from church, or other relative who can. If these options are not available to you, you may want to consider hiring a geriatric care manager. These professionals are typically nurses or social workers and can be hired on a fee-for-service basis to provide a wide range of support and care services. They can be knowledgeable about health-care resources, serve as your "eyes and ears" in the hospital while you are unavailable, and be an invaluable advocate for your loved one's needs.

Step 2: Connect with the Professionals

Healthcare is like many other things in life: a personal relationship and good rapport can make everything go a bit more smoothly. Learn to communicate well with the professionals involved in your loved one's care and keep focused on the needs of your loved one. Keep the staff aware of how to best contact you to make sure you are kept up-to-date on your loved one's condition. A word of caution: don't get caught in the HIPAA (Health Insurance Portability and Accountability Act) roadblock. HIPPA is a federal law which may prevent healthcare providers from disclosing information to you about your loved one's condition. Make sure you are listed as someone who can receive information. Most often, a medical release, such as a living will or durable power of attorney for health care, signed by your loved one, will be needed to allow health care providers to deliver information about his or her health status to you. If there is no such formal document, some health care settings will accept a verbal release from your loved one.

Step 3: Learn the Facts and the Options

Leeza: Anne Marie did the initial wave of research to find the right people and places, so we could take Mom in to be tested. I flew home to get the diagnosis and we were all there together. It was a life changing moment. It was enormously comforting to Mom to have us all there, I think. It also gave the medical team more of a sense of urgency having the entire family there, and we were all able to get the same information at the same time. Whenever possible, we tried very hard to hear information as a group.

We also spoke with a social worker and a geriatrician the day we got the diagnosis. Afterwards, we all took Mom to lunch, ignoring the hole in our hearts and assuring Mom that we were lucky because her disease was caught early. We told her there were meds now that weren't available before; that it wasn't going to be like it had been with Granny. And all that was true. Mom was put on Aricept right away along with some nutritional supplements and shortly afterwards, she was put on anti-depressants, which helped a lot. We were so grateful for the Aricept because it gave Mom something to focus on, it allowed her feel that she was being pro-active with her care, and it did steady her symptoms for about two years after that. I gave her daily pep talks with my best optimistic delivery. I will never regret staying hopeful. I don't think it's being naïve or having your head in the sand, I think it's essential to stay focused on the promise of possibility because it's always there.

When we finally got a diagnosis, when we finally knew what we were up against, we each gave what we had. Carl had his legal expertise. He knew how to protect Mom's property. He knew how to make sure we had a living will and a durable power of attorney. Cammy was physically available. She was the one who was most present to check on Mom and look after Dad. Anne Marie was "command central" for resources. Typically she would do the research, about the disease, about treatment, and then communicate it to me and I would follow up. My job was to keep everything moving. Pushing forward, trying something new, coming around the corner and through the back door and staying positive, at least on the surface. I think being the middle child allowed me to more easily look at all sides of things.

Too often, the overwhelming newness and complexity of the healthcare system causes us to become passive. Sometimes it's easier to simply accept the advice and opinions given to us by the professionals. But in some instances, they offer only routine suggestions. Be proactive. Ask them if there are any alternatives available. As examples: can rehabilitation be provided in my mother's home instead of in a hospital? What would we need to do to have her go home?

What do the different facilities available for this kind of care offer? Is there a superior facility across town for this type of problem? Often, patients are referred to care facilities based upon the assumption that the patient prefers to be close to home. If you are willing to go where the care for the type of problem being faced is best, let that be known. It might be the place down the street, but it might be an hour away. Being open to finding the most skilled and successful providers of the type of care you need will serve you well.

Leeza: Expect to be overwhelmed when dealing with the medical community. It's not that the doctors are doing anything wrong, necessarily; it's just that it's their routine, but it's your living hell. I remember being a little angry during Mom's appointments and upset with Dad if he wasn't being as revealing as I thought he should be about how bad Mom's condition was. I would get angry during phone conversations with the doctors if they didn't treat my mother the way I thought she deserved. I would sometimes get agitated and frustrated. Remember, take a friend with you, make notes or record the visit on a mini-recorder because chances are you are not going to remember everything that is said. Print out a list of questions beforehand and take them with you. If you are lucky enough to have a "team" with you, each of you could take a different role (as questioner, as note taker) when you go.

The one area where my siblings and I often traded roles was being the shoulder to cry on and being the one who needed to cry. We are so blessed that we are all so close. Cammy and I spent a lot of time on the phone. Sometimes those calls were the only things that kept me sane. I also talked a lot on the phone with Mom trying desperately to stay in the moment and hang onto every last piece of her. Daddy's role?

Well, Dad was shell-shocked and yet he went through the mo-tions of the dutiful husband and was patient and consistent. I believe these might have been things he was not able to give Mom earlier in their marriage because of his work. But I think he really treasured being in a position where she needed him because Mom had always been so independent.

Step 4: Plan Ahead

Always look down the road and plan for the next steps. Tomorrow will come more quickly than you think, and you do not want to be forced to make hasty decisions. This can be challenging when the next steps are not entirely clear. But even if all the details of the type of care that is needed are not yet fully known, you can often get a lot done ahead of time. For example, if you know your loved one will need continued care at another facility once she is discharged, review the financial resources available and if appropriate, discuss her preferences for the type of facility and its location. Clear up differences of opinion within the family about this issue before you have to make the final decisions. You can then narrow down the options as your loved one's health status and her "next-step" needs become clearer.

Step 5: Stay Calm and Focused - No Matter What They Throw at You

A typical caregiver lament is, "I never knew one day to the next what was coming... I wanted to walk away." The best course of action to avoid feeling this way is to keep yourself focused on the key outcomes for your loved one. Is the goal to get to rehabilitation? Is the goal to get back home? Is the goal to have your loved one free of pain? Keep the answers to these questions in mind and remind the professional care team of them, directly and often, if you see they are moving in a direction away from your overall goals.

For any caregiver, the stress level is enormous. You must be prepared and steel yourself to stay calm, get the facts, and deal with whatever arises. At times, there is no room for emotion; often, emotion must wait until after the decisions are made. And to make good decisions, you need to have good information. The professionals don't always recognize the caregiver's need for information, so caregivers must ask for it. Medical professionals are very busy, and you may have to ask two or three times, but so be it. Never raise your voice, never be mean, but be persistent.

Step 6: Reach Out For Help From The Community

Anne Marie: When Jean began having symptoms, none of us had had any firsthand knowledge of or experience with Alzheimer's disease in a person as young as she. I don't ever recall Jean ever describing any of the behaviors her mother exhibited, so we didn't know what to look for in Jean, any time that Carlos and I visited Jean's mother in the nursing home, she was either asleep or silent, so we never had any interaction with her or observed any of the behaviors of an Alzheimer's disease patient.

Over time, We all recognized that she was getting forgetful and repeating herself, but I think we assumed that is was a natural part of the aging process, or perhaps she was having a glass of wine too many in the afternoon. It was only after the behaviors continued and became more pronounced that we honestly considered (or admitted to ourselves) that she might really have dementia.

Being a lifetime resident of Columbia and very involved

in the community, I became the researcher (my natural instinct!). Not only was this a good task for me, but as close as we all are, and as close as I was to Jean, this process seemed so intimate and personal that at the time I felt that only the immediate family should be with Jean as they went through the incredibly frightening, unfamiliar process of diagnosis and making the enormous decisions about her future. I felt it more appropriate for me to gather information and help guide the process. I talked to people who had relatives with AD, physicians, hospital staff and the Alzheimer's Association (the only "specialized" AD organization in South Carolina at the time) to try to understand the disease, how to treat it, and where to find professional help. I have to say, it was not an easy task. I was amazed at the lack of understanding, information and resources available for learning about AD and finding appropriate care for AD patients. I remember that the materials we collected from outside sources, both from the standpoint of the information that was given and the quality of the resources available, were completely unverified, which disturbed me a great deal. What a difference a decade makes!

I spoke several times with an acquaintance who was a nurse and social worker for a geriatric physicians' office and a neurologist she knew before I felt I had some degree of understanding about how to navigate our way through this. Having gleaned as much as I could from reliable resources, I had many conversations with Leeza to share what we had learned and make a plan with the rest of the family.

Caregiving is an enormous task that is too much for just one individual, or even one family, to handle without support. Community resources are invaluable for strengthening your caregiving family, helping you through crises, or just providing a much needed respite from the daily burdens you face.

Begin researching the assistance resources available in your area while the disease is still in its early stages. Services are often available from voluntary organizations, religious groups and governmental agencies. Places to begin your investigation include:

- Your healthcare professionals.
- Local chapters of national organizations such as the Alzheimer's Association.
- Federal government agencies on aging.
- State and county government programs.
- Community hotlines.
- National links and referral services, such as the Alzheimer's Disease Education and Referral Center.

For a valuable list of resources you can call upon for information and help, please visit the Resources section at the end of this book.

As the disorder progresses, you will need to call upon more and more resources to help care for your loved one. Having the information on hand well before you need it eases stress and provides a quick helping hand if you begin to get overwhelmed. For example, if the phone number for the local Alzheimer's Resource Center is on hand and you already know that they offer caregiver support groups, you are more likely to go than if you had to search for the information in the middle of overwhelming stress at home.

Leeza's Place offers a number of programs to assist caregivers and their loved ones deal with the challenges of a memory loss disorder. For example, in partnership with the Alzheimer's Association, its offers E.A.S.E., the Early Alzheimer's Support and Education Program for the recently diagnosed that focuses on educating about

Carlos, Sr.'s 02 for Caregivers

DON'T GET OVERWHELMED

Emotional exhaustion comes at you slowly over time, but physical exhaustion hits you like a ton of bricks. When the two combined, I just did not know how to carry on. If this is how you feel then:

- Ask for and accept help.
- Consider respite care for yourself. You deserve a break!
- Know your limits. Don't let guilt restrict your ability to say no.
- Talk! Join a support group for caregivers, see a therapist or confide in a trusted friend.
- Find time for yourself and take it one day at a time. Recognize that you will have good days and bad days.

treatment, expected complications, and care-related skills development. It also offers the Lunch and Learn Caregiver Skills Seminars, an educational program covering topics including legal and financial issues. The Caring for the Caregiver educational series provides information on the physical and emotional aspects of caregiving, and the Bereavement Support Program aims to assist caregivers experiencing the loss of a loved one.

Finding Help - The Payoff

"I was glad I had the family around me to help find good care for Jean," Carlos, Sr. recalls. "Cammy and Anne Marie were never afraid to ask questions, and once we found doctors we trusted, it was a huge weight off all of our shoulders."

When caregivers are asked who they can count on to listen to and understand their questions and concerns and then render valuable medical opinions, unfortunately the answer is all too often, "no one." If you find yourself in that situation, resist the understandable urge to run away! Return to Step 1. Listen and learn your loved one's needs and desires. Persistently seek advice and answers from the professionals you encounter. Don't stop until you find someone who will both listen and advise, in that order. Be prepared. You, your loved one and your family will be glad you did. And remember, the moment you've reached out and connected with that first resource for information or help, you've taken one of your first and most important breaths of that all-important oxygen.

PART II:

CARING FOR THE CAREGIVER'S BODY

Happiness lies, first of all, in health.

—George William Curtis

CHAPTER 4

The Benefits of Exercise

Carlos, Sr.: When Jean's illness caught up with us, I was at an age when I didn't think physical fitness was so important anymore. Boy, was I wrong! One day I was taking her for a walk by the lake and she slipped and fell. I could barely help her up, and in trying I wrenched my back pretty badly. So bad, in fact, that I couldn't even do the simplest tasks for her – or myself – for a few weeks. Later, when Cammy moved in, I started paying better attention to my physical fitness. I wish I hadn't waited so long.

Caregiving is a tough business! It requires tremendous reserves of physical strength and stamina. As caregivers, we need to keep up with our own daily tasks, be physically able to help our loved ones as they lose the ability to help themselves, and be able to stay active throughout the day and often throughout much of the night. Over time, the physical demands of caregiving can put caregivers at greater risk than the average person for illness, chronic fatigue and emotional stress. Because of this, physical fitness is especially critical for caregivers. In this and the following chapter we'll examine the challenges caregiving can place on your body, and we'll lay out simple steps you can follow to ensure that you are physically strong enough to handle these challenges without losing your own health.

First, what is good health? In a survey performed by Harvard University, an amazing 95% of respondents defined good health as being "when there is an absence of pain." But good health isn't just a *lack* of something. Instead, it is a positive state, one in which we are not only free of disease but full of life energy. The World Health Organization defines health as "a state of complete physical, mental and social well-being and not merely the absence of disease or infirmity." By this definition, good health means possessing mental and physical well-being and a strong social connection with others.

Good health starts with good *physical* health. What concrete actions can you take to improve your physical health in the midst of your busy caregiving life? The hardest part is committing to make your physical health a priority. Once you've taken this important first step, the path to overall good health and vitality is simply about learning what to do and how to do it, and having fun along the way.

How Exercise Helps Us

The most effective medication for many ailments isn't medication at all—it's simple exercise! Exercise is the key to preventing much of the extra wear and tear we experience as caregivers, and it provides us with the energy to handle our work without becoming ill. Incorporating physical exercise into your daily routine has many benefits that include lowering blood pressure, raising *high-density lipoprotein* (good cholesterol) levels and lowering *low-density lipoprotein* (bad cholesterol) levels, as well as improving blood flow throughout the body and increasing the heart's working capacity. Conditions such as diabetes and arthritis can be managed, at least in part, by regular exercise. With exercise, your bones can rebuild and repair themselves instead of becoming thin and porous, a condition known as *osteoporosis*. In some cases, exercise can actually eliminate the need for costly medications, which means no more unpleasant drug side effects.

New medical research suggests that physical exercise also encourages healthy brains to function at optimum levels (see Chapter 6, Brain Fitness and Sleep). Fitness prompts nerve cells to multiply, strengthens their connections with each other, and protects them from harm. Exercise also positively affects our emotions: during exercise, the brain increases the production of hormones known as *endorphins*, which help to elevate mood and reduce feelings of fatigue. In other words, exercise can help us feel happier and calmer. Exercising regularly also helps relieve stress and increase mental clarity because it provides a way for the body to release tension and pent-up frustration.

Exercising doesn't need to be excessively strenuous, complicated, or time consuming. Thirty minutes of moderate activity a day is the goal. For some, spending this amount of time exercising each day is simply not possible, but that's okay. Studies have shown that ten-minutes bursts of moderate activity done on a regular basis, can make a difference, and this can include activities that are a part of your normal routine. The point is anyone and everyone can increase his or her activity level in some way. Throw out your excuses and open yourself up to the benefits of exercise!

Getting Started

Once you've made the commitment to good health, it's time to make sure that you choose a plan of exercise that is right for you, one that you will enjoy and stay with over the long term. Consider the following steps in creating a successful and enjoyable exercise plan. Remember, just take one extra step each day and you'll find yourself moving forward. It's easier than you think.

Step 1: Talk to your doctor, especially if you have been physi-

WHEN THE CAREGIVER GETS SICK

Caregiving is a chronically stressful activity that can compromise the immune system and lead to physical illness. While elderly caregivers who experience caregiver-related stress have a 63% higher mortality rate than their non-caregiver peers, they are also known to follow preventive health care advice less often than people who are not caregivers.

For illnesses such as colds and the flu, do what you've always done: get more sleep, increase your fluid intake and eat sensibly. Take medications to relieve symptoms and consider relaxing activities such as a long bath or a foot massage. If you suffer severe symptoms or symptoms that you have not had before, make an appointment with your physician for an evaluation.

Recovering from a minor illness is very important, but how you take care of yourself afterwards is equally important. Learn the lesson of the illness and do what you can to help your body recover fully and become stronger than it was before you became ill. Remember, you may be facing a decade of giving care to your loved one, so you need to have plans in place to stay strong over the long term. Keep your stress levels under control with frequent relaxation, go to the doctor as often as you should, and don't ignore the symptoms of illnesses that need attention.

For those suffering from chronic ailments such as high blood pressure, diabetes, arthritis, and heart and lung disease who may find it difficult to regularly follow their doctors' advice about diet, exercise or other therapies, each of these illnesses can be improved by "taking your oxygen first":

- Locate respite care for your loved one so you can go to the doctor, plan meals, and exercise.
- Make sure your doctor knows that you are a caregiver. He or she can then consider this when caring for you.
- Find a mail-order pharmacy or one that emphasizes customer service to avoid the risk of running out of medications or to decrease your time waiting in line.
- Speak with a nutritionist about meal planning for both you and your loved one.

You don't have to be a caregiver to want to avoid a mammogram, a colonoscopy, a dental checkup or a flu vaccine! But don't you use that excuse. More than anyone else, caregivers need to stay on top of their preventive health measures. This type of care focuses on preventing cancer and infection, and over the long course of caring for someone with a memory loss disorder, caregivers are at increased risk for both. The type of preventive care you need will depend on your age, personal health status and medical history. Making an appointment with your doctor to specifically discuss preventative care is another way to ensure your general health and well being.

cally inactive for some time or have any chronic illnesses. Let your doctor know your plans and make sure you are able to meet the demands of the plan you have chosen.

Step 2: Choose activities that you will enjoy. If you can't bring yourself to continue with the exercises you choose, you will not reap their benefits. Think about the kinds of physical activities you enjoy: perhaps walking, swimming, tennis, dancing, or gardening. Remember to keep it fun! Investigate the exercise programs that are available in your area at senior centers, at your local Leeza's Place or YWCA. Decide if you wish to exercise independently, "one on one" with a trainer, or in a class.

Step 3: Be realistic in your expectations. Increase your exercise time slowly. For example, if you choose to walk for exercise, perhaps start with just a short walk around the yard before progressing to a walk around the block. Start with small increments of gentle activity, and then increase as you feel stronger. Be aware of any discomfort or signs of overexertion, such as dizziness, and talk to your doctor if this happens. Drink plenty of water as you exercise, especially if the weather is warm, and avoid outdoor activities when the temperature outside is extremely warm or cold.

Step 4: Keep track of your progress. Studies show that if you keep a daily log of your activity, you will be more likely to keep up with it. You might designate an area in a journal or create a separate log book for just that purpose.

What Kind of Exercise Should You Do?

Keep in mind that your plan should incorporate exercises that work to enhance your *endurance*, your *strength*, your *balance* and your *flexibility*.

Endurance relates to one's overall physical condition; it is the ability to exert oneself for an extended period without growing fatigued. While typical endurance-type exercises include running, swimming and bicycling, you can increase your physical endurance with any exercise as you gradually work to increase the length of time you do it.

Strength exercises build muscle, and strong muscles increase the amount of force one can exert for a given task. When you have strong muscles, you can get up from a chair by yourself, you can lift your grandchildren, and you can walk through the park. Keeping your muscles in shape helps prevent falls, which avoids problems such as broken hips. Consider adding weight lifting to your routine. You need not use excessive weight or go out and buy dumbbells; even using a bottle of water and doing arm lifts while watching the news can be helpful.

Balance is the ability to maintain your center of gravity and avoid falls. Strengthening the lower body muscles leads to greater stability and fewer falls. *Flexibility* involves freeing the range of your physical motion, making it easier for you to reach down to tie your shoes or look over your shoulder when you back the car out of the driveway. The following chart can help you chose the exercise that is best for you:

Exercise Classes

Many people enjoy exercise classes for the chance to learn something new and to enjoy the support of the group. There are many available, from ballroom dancing to bicycle spin classes. Options such as *tai chi*, *yoga* and *water exercises* are particularly good because they can help with strength, flexibility and balance, and are especially helpful for relieving stress and learning to settle the mind.

EXERCISE	Endurance	Strength	Balance	Flexibility
Walking	✗	✗	✗	✗
WATER-BASED *Lap Swimming* *Waterobics* *Water Walking*	✗		✗	✗
Tai Chi, Yoga			✗	✗
Free Weights		✗		
Chair Exercises		✗	✗	✗
NuStep *Treadmills* *Cardio Machines*	✗	✗	✗	

TAI CHI

Tai chi literally means "moving life force". This ancient form of exercise is becoming more and more popular because it is a gentle workout that leaves you feeling energized. Tai chi challenges the mind as well as the body and is especially effective at reducing stress.

Tai chi combines routines of deep breathing, posturing, stretching, swaying, and other controlled movements with meditation. The clothing is "come as you are" and people of every size, shape, age, and fitness level participate. A typical tai chi class progressively introduces the movements of a tai chi form. You will gradually be introduced to more movements until you are accomplished in the entire series, much like learning the steps of a dance. You'll note that no one seems to be exerting himself. Is this really exercise? You bet. And, by moving through its series of choreographed movements very slowly and in a state of absolute relaxation, you are virtually forced to let go of grudges, resentments, and anything that keeps you from connecting with your body. Tai chi provides all of the positive aspects of aerobic activity, such as increasing heart strength and overall energy. Researchers have also found that tai chi, with its emphasis on balance and controlled movements, decreases the incidence of the number of falls suffered by its practitioners, with some studies reporting a reduction by as much as fifty percent! Another benefit of tai chi is increased blood circulation, which seems to help alleviate the pains of arthritis.

Tai chi is offered through private instruction, classes, books, and video. Classes can be found through community centers, senior centers, health clubs, or hospital-sponsored programs. If you are thinking of joining a class, ask questions of the instructor and participants to make sure it's the right one for you: how long has the instructor been teaching? Do the other students like the class? What keeps them coming back? Take a "test class" or two, if possible. Most instructors allow you to visit or sample a class free or for a minimal charge before joining. It's important that you feel comfortable with the teacher and like his or her style.

YOGA

Yoga unifies the body, mind and spirit and is a path to personal growth and healing. Its goal is to reach complete peace in body and mind. There are many forms of yoga, each with a different focus. Some forms, like Hatha yoga, are more concerned with postures and breathing exercises, and focus more on spirituality. Others, like Ashtanga or power yoga, are more physically demanding. If you are interested in simply increasing physical health and reducing stress, Hatha yoga is probably right for you; it's more gentle and appropriate for all levels of fitness. Yoga helps tone and strengthen muscles, increases flexibility and encourages deep, even breathing. Studies have shown that it can relieve the symptoms of several common illnesses such as arthritis, arteriosclerosis, chronic fatigue, diabetes, asthma and obesity. Like tai chi, yoga incorporates meditation for reducing stress and increasing everyday awareness of our bodies. A typical class begins with easy stretching and relaxing breathing techniques. Students are instructed in various physical poses which vary in degree of difficulty. An experienced instructor can tailor poses to your own personal abilities and limitations. Movements are typically slow and the class is quiet or accompanied by soft music to encourage a meditative state.

Yoga is now available nearly everywhere, from gyms and special yoga centers to community centers and even hospitals. You can also find guidance from videos and books, which makes at-home learning easier, although you miss out on the feedback and sociability of a class. As with other exercise programs you may be considering, ask questions in advance. Is the class suitable for a beginner? Is the instructor knowledgeable about health conditions such as joint or back problems? Can he or she modify poses for you to prevent injury?

WATER EXERCISE

Water exercise makes for a terrific workout for nearly anyone, of any age and fitness level. Compared to exercising on land, water offers more resistance than air to your muscles, which also have to work against the body's natural tendency to float in the water, creating a harder workout. Other benefits of water exercise include the ability to extend the limbs farther while underwater, increasing the range of motion (particularly good for arthritis); a decreased risk of injury from falling; and less stress on the joints. New research also indicates that water exercise may be effective in fighting osteoporosis.

As with any form of exercise, you will need to take some common-sense precautions: don't swim alone; use a flotation belt if there is a chance you can end up in deep water and your swimming skills are limited; stay hydrated; and wear water shoes to improve traction on the floor of the pool.

Exercising With Your Loved One

You need not exercise alone. Just as we can benefit from exercise, so too can those with Alzheimer's disease and other disorders. It may take a little imagination to find activities both of you are challenged by and can enjoy, but shared exercise can be a very welcome break from the daily "do this, do that" of caregiving and a way to enjoy each other's company when conversation is limited.

Exercising together can be incorporated into your daily caregiving routine. Gardening, walking the dog, pushing the wheelchair around the block or picking up trash can all be done as a duo. The easiest, safest, and most readily available physical activity for a person with a memory disorder is walking with someone else. You can take your loved one to the safe, climate controlled environment of a shopping mall; many malls have "mall-walking" programs that offer structure, incentives, and social opportunities. Such programs are perfect for an accompanied person with dementia. Other activities include hiking, dancing, tandem cycling, boating and household tasks. In addition to being an enjoyable way to spend time together while increasing your physical fitness, studies show that exercise reduces the frequency of unwanted behaviors such as wandering, pulling at clothing, making repetitive noises, swearing and aggressive acts, as well as improving communication and social participation.

Avoiding Physical Injury While Caregiving

The two main areas at greatest risk for injury from the typical caregiving activities are the lower back and the arms and shoulders. For the caregiver in particular, there are two specific areas of improvement you should strive for if you are going to be responsible for the physical care of a loved one. The first is *proper body mechanics*, and the second is strengthening the back, shoulder and neck muscles.

BODY MECHANICS

Body mechanics refers to the way in which we move our bodies. It involves standing and moving in ways that prevent injury, avoid fatigue, and make the best use of one's strength when performing physical tasks. When you learn how to move, control and balance your own body, it's easier to move another person. Here are some of the basics of proper body mechanics for lifting:

- Only lift as much as you can comfortably handle.
- Always let the person you are helping know what you are going to do.
- Plan the lift—check the area for slippery spots or possible tripping hazards. (Wearing non-skid heels and soles will be safer for both you and the person you are assisting).
- To create a base of support for the task at hand, stand with your

GAIT BELTS

Gait belts are specifically designed to aid in moving people with mobility issues. Worn by the loved one, they help give caregivers a firmer grip while assisting a loved to move about the home. When you are helping someone walk, use one hand to firmly hold the gait belt (or waistband if you are not using a gait belt.) If there is no waistband, you will need to use two hands, with one placed on the shoulder and the other hand placed on the opposite hip. In the event of a fall, gait belts help the caregiver to lift the loved one with decreased risk of injury to herself.

feet 8"–12" apart with one foot a half step ahead of the other.
- Bend your knees slightly.
- Keep your spine in a neutral (normal arched, not stiff) position while lifting.
- Before starting to move someone, count with the person, "1-2-3."
- Lift with the legs, not with the back.

Special Caregiver Needs: Strengthening the Back, Neck and Shoulder Muscles

Caregivers are especially susceptible to injuries to the back, neck and shoulders. The following exercises should be performed as part of what we call the *Caregiver's Exercise Circuit*. This is about ten minutes of exercises that focus on flexibility and strengthening of the back, neck, and shoulders. Do these once a day and you'll stay strong in these critical areas and protect yourself from injury.

THE CAREGIVER'S EXERCISE CIRCUIT

Do all of the following exercises 10 times. Extend only as far as you can comfortably stretch.

BACK STRENGTHENING EXERCISES

Knee Lifts

Lie on your back on your bed or the floor with your knees bent and the soles of your feet flat on the bed or floor. Use your arms to hug one knee at a time to your chest. Repeat ten times for each knee. Then lift both knees to your chest at the same time and repeat this move ten times.

Abdominal Crunches

Lie on your back on your bed or the floor with your knees bent and soles on the bed/floor. Gently raise your chest so your shoulders come off the bed or floor. You should feel your abdominal muscles tighten. Repeat 10 times.

Hip Extensions

Lie on your stomach on your bed or the floor with your legs straight out behind you. Tighten your buttock muscles first and then lift one leg about 4-8 inches. Keep your knee straight. Hold for 5 seconds. Then lower your leg and relax. Repeat with the opposite leg. Do each leg 10 times.

NECK AND SHOULDER EXERCISES

Arms Overhead

Lie on your back on your bed or the floor. Slowly bring your arms straight up. Keep your hands about 6 inches apart and the elbows straight. Let your arms fall slowly down behind your head as far as you can. Slowly return your arms to your sides. Repeat 10 times.

Neck Rolls

While lying in bed or on the floor, roll your head from side to side by bending your neck so your right ear points towards the right shoulder, dropping your chin to your chest, then bending to the left so the left ear points to the left shoulder and then returning the head to center. Try to go as far as you can in each direction without pain. Don't let the shoulders creep up toward the ears. Do this 10 times.

Shoulder Lifts

Slowly lift both shoulders up toward your ears. Try to lift them as high as they will go. Repeat this exercise 10 times.

Shoulder Circles

Slowly roll your shoulders forward as far as they can go. From that forward position, lift the shoulders up toward your ears as far as they will go and then back as far as they will go so that you form circles from front to rear. Do this 10 times. Repeat the shoulder rolls starting from the rear and going to the front. Do this 10 times.

What Keeps You From Working Out?

Having trouble getting started with your exercise program, or keeping up with it? Be honest with yourself about why you're avoiding exercise. If there is a physical reason, go to the doctor and get your health in order so that you can maintain your fitness level. If you simply don't like exercising, you need to think about ways to increase your daily activities. Try more vacuuming! Window shop *before* filling your cart! If a lack of time is the problem, you can work towards three 10- minute exercise sessions instead of a longer session. If it's the cost, you can set up a walking plan and some exercises at home and avoid the fees charged by the gym. If your caregiving duties keep you from leaving your loved one, consider ways to exercise together.

Physical Fitness - The Payoff

Carlos, Sr. remembers, "Starting to pay attention to my fitness was one of the best investments I ever made, and it paid off for Jean as well as for me. It helped me sleep better, I had fewer aches and pains, and I had lots more energy for things like walks to the lake (and back!)."

Remember, it's never too late (or too difficult) to get into better physical shape. Increasing endurance, strength, flexibility and balance, and using good body mechanics, rank high among the useful tools for protecting your health and well being. With your extra strength and flexibility, you'll have fewer aches and pains from your difficult caregiving chores. You'll have greater endurance to get you through the many tasks you'll face. And you'll feel a greater sense of vitality and energy that affect all you do.

But as you work through the Three E's, Energizing yourself doesn't just come from building your muscles and increasing your flexibility. Your *whole self* must become as healthy as possible. That includes proper feeding of not only your body but your mind and spirit. In the next chapters we'll examine how your journey through the Three E's, and through the caregiving experience, will make you stronger in ways you may never have imagined.

CHAPTER 5

Eating Well

*C*ammy: *Growing up, our lives revolved around the family meals. I remember Mom planning lunch at breakfast and dinner at lunch. Dad was born, bred and wed on typical southern cuisine – lots of fried anything and casseroles loaded with cheese and topped with Ritz crackers. Sweet iced tea was always around, too. Not regular sweetened tea, but really more like a ton of sugar with a bit of tea and lemon flavor.*

Mom and Dad were also what I think of as a bit more than social drinkers. A favorite expression in our house was "When the sun goes down, it's time to go brown," meaning, after 5 o'clock, it was O.K. to move on to bourbon cocktails.

I wasn't aware of the toll caring for Mom had taken on Dad until I moved from Los Angeles back home after we had to move Mom to the assisted living facility. He had lost a lot of weight. Mom had always been the cook in the house and after she fell ill Dad simply wasn't eating. He was also drinking more; with the stresses of caring for Mom, it was quicker and easier for him to grab a drink than to prepare a meal, and his health began to suffer. His body was telling him the calories he got from that drink should be coming from more nutritious foods. I made sure that Dad started eating three meals a day again, but I served meals that included a lot less meat, fat and sugar and a lot more fruits and vegetables than my Dad was used to. While Dad complained about my "California cooking," I am pretty sure it is what saved him from having a heart attack.

What is Nutrition?

Nutrition refers to the intake of *nutrients,* such as carbohydrates, fats, protein, water, vitamins and minerals that allow the body to grow and to repair itself. Without proper nutrition, bodily processes, such as creating energy and ridding the body of waste, do not function adequately, and can eventually lead to serious health problems. Getting proper nutrition while giving care to a loved one is often difficult; in some cases, the pressures of caregiving make it difficult to find the time to plan, prepare and eat meals regularly. For Carlos, Sr., poor nutrition took over until his daughter Cammy assumed responsibility for preparing the family meals. He also fell into the habit, common among caregivers, of drinking more alcohol than he normally would, which blunts the appetite for nutrient-rich food. Combined, these changes led to weight loss, a visible indication of his caregiver stress. But keep in mind that not everyone who is poorly nourished will suffer a visible weight change. In some cases, weight may appear normal or even ideal but nutritional quality is lacking. Nutrition and weight are not the same thing. While our society places tremendous emphasis on weight, overall nutritional status is most important. Even those who are underweight or ideal weight can suffer the effects of malnutrition due to poor food selection.

Many caregivers are unaware of their risk for poor nutrition. An easy way to determine the state of your nutritional well being is to take the following test. If any of the following statements describes you, give yourself the number of points indicated:

- An illness or condition has caused you to change the amount or kind of food you eat = 2 points
- Most days you eat fewer than two meals = 3 points
- You eat few fruits, vegetable, or dairy products = 2 points
- You have three or more servings of beer, wine, or liquor most days = 2 points
- You have tooth or mouth problems that make it hard to eat = 2 points
- You don't always have enough money to buy healthy foods = 4 points
- You eat alone most of the time = 1point
- You take three of more prescription drugs or over the counter drugs each day = 1 point
- Without wanting to, you have lost or gained ten pounds in the last six months = 2 points
- You are not always physically able to shop, cook, or feed yourself = 2 points*

A score of zero to two points puts you at a low risk for poor nutrition, three to five points puts you at a moderately high risk, while six points or more means you are at a high risk for poor nutrition. If you are at moderate or high risk for poor nutrition, you need to make changes in your diet.

What is a Healthy Diet?

The Center for Nutrition Policy and Promotion, an agency of the United States Department of Agriculture (U.S.D.A.) publishes die-

---

* *The Nutrition Screening Initiative, 2005.* A project of the American Academy of Family Physicians, The American Diabetic Association and the National Council on the Aging, Inc.

tary guidelines that describe a healthy diet as one emphasizing fruits, vegetables, whole grains and fat-free or low-fat milk and milk products and includes lean meats, poultry, fish, beans, eggs, and nuts. It is low in saturated fats, *transfats*, cholesterol, salt and added sugars. We'll discuss some of these in detail later in this chapter. An excellent resource for assessing your diet and creating a healthful diet that is right for you is the U.S.D.A.'s website, www.mypyramid.gov. You can complete an assessment of the nutritional components in your current diet and make menus that will improve your dietary intake.

A Word About Water

Drinking water is one of the most effective means of ensuring good health. Water maintains and regulates the body's systems and acts as a preventative measure against common disorders and illness. Our bodies use water for digestion, to absorb nutrients, for blood circulation and for excreting waste. Water is a vital nutrient that the body cannot store for later use. That is why we need to constantly replenish our bodies' supply. To avoid dehydration, the body needs a minimum of eight eight-ounce glasses of water daily. The precise amount you need depends on your level of activity, the outside temperature and humidity level, your medications, illnesses and the other foods you eat. Remember, if you are exercising, your daily need for water will increase.

Normally, about 20% of the water we take in every day comes from food, while the rest comes from drinking water and beverages. But be wary of caffeinated beverages: they can act as a bladder irritant and diuretic, causing increased urination and water loss. Try to balance your caffeinated beverage intake by drinking an equal amount of water during the day. If you find it hard to drink enough water each day, consider eating foods with higher water content,

DEHYDRATION AND SENIOR CAREGIVERS

A number of changes in the aging body can lead to dehydration becoming particularly dangerous to seniors. First, the thirst mechanisms and reflexes are diminished such that the drive to drink is reduced. The ability to sweat and cool the body is also diminished and leads to increased body temperature, especially in hot climates. In older adults, the heart is more dependent on blood volume to achieve good blood circulation. Dehydration lowers the volume of blood circulating in the body and can lead to decreased blood flow to all the organs but especially the kidneys, the ability of which to concentrate and conserve water diminishes in older persons. Taken together, the state of dehydration is a dangerous one for the aging body and it is especially important for the older person to keep up his or her fluid intake.

such as fruits. Always avoid drinking water at the beginning of meals, as it works to suppress the appetite.

Fruits and Vegetables

An important point to make about this food category is that one cannot be substituted for the other. The guidelines indicate that a healthy diet includes five servings a day of *both* fruits and vegetables. There is a tendency among many to eat more fruits instead of vegetables, and only five instead of ten servings. Also be aware that, while your mother may have a different opinion on this, there is really very little difference in the nutritional quality of fruits and vegetables that are eaten raw or eaten cooked. Fresh, frozen, canned or dried; whole, cut-up, or mashed, they are all virtually the same. The important thing is that getting ten servings, no matter how you slice it, is the goal.

Whole Grains

Grains can be either *refined* or *whole*. Refined grains have been milled and no longer contain the bran or germ which contain dietary fiber, iron, and many B vitamins. Consuming foods rich in fiber, such as whole grains, reduces the risk of coronary heart disease and may reduce constipation. Whole grains are also low on the *glycemic index*, a measurement of how foods affect our blood sugar levels. Foods with a high glycemic index cause blood glucose levels to surge quickly. Over time, the steady ingestion of foods high on the glycemic index may lead to a greater risk of developing diabetes and heart disease. In general, whole grains have a much lower glycemic index than refined grains. They have the added benefit of being able to help you lose weight.

Obviously, the healthiest choice is whole grains, and at least half of our daily grain consumption should be whole grains. Examples of whole grains include whole wheat flour, bulgur (cracked wheat), brown rice, oatmeal, cornmeal and popcorn. Choose foods that list these ingredients first on the label's ingredient list. "Multi-grain," "stone-ground," "100% wheat," "cracked wheat," "seven-grain," or "bran" are usually *not* whole-grain products. Also, the color of food does not guarantee that it contains whole grains: bread can be brown because of the addition of molasses or other ingredients. Read the ingredient list to make sure you are buying a whole grain product.

Dietary Oils

There has been much debate over how much fat is necessary for health. The question now is really better phrased as, "What *kind* of fats are necessary for good health?" The answer is *monounsaturated* or *polyunsaturated fats*, both of which are commonly found in vegetable oils, which are considered liquid fats. Fats in solid form, such as butter or margarine, contain more *saturated fats* and/or *trans fats* than oils. Saturated fats, trans fats, and cholesterol tend to raise LDL ("bad") cholesterol levels in the blood, which in turn increases the risk for heart disease. No plant oils contain cholesterol, but a few plant oils, such as coconut oil and palm kernel oil, are high in saturated fats and for nutritional purposes should be considered solid fats.

It's important to include enough of the "good" fats in your diet. Polyunsaturated fats contain *fatty acids* essential to our well being (called "essential fatty acids"). The fats found in fish, such as salmon, trout and herring, nuts, flax seeds and vegetable oils including corn, canola and olive oil do not raise LDL ("bad") cholesterol levels in the blood. In addition to providing essential fatty acids, oils are the major source of vitamin E in typical American diets.

Foods that contain the "bad", saturated fats include coconut oil, palm oil and cocoa butter. Equally important is to avoid as much as possible foods containing transfats: French fries, doughnuts, cookies, muffins, pies and cakes all are high in transfats. Generally, commercially fried and baked goods found in fast food restaurants, containing a great deal of transfats. While it's not a good idea to make any fats a large part of your diet, it is better to have good fats than none at all.

What's the Skinny on Diets?

Buyer beware! If "diets" worked, there wouldn't be so many. But it seems that every day there's another "miracle" diet product or the "best diet ever" on the market. From a nutritional standpoint, however, one diet to keep in mind as you plan your menus is the "Mediterranean diet", a meal plan based on the kinds and quantities of foods traditionally eaten by those living in Greece and Southern Italy, who experience much lower rates of cardiovascular and other diseases than does the American population. Not so much a fad diet as a lifestyle diet, it has attributes that are very similar to the U.S.D.A. recommendations. It also avoids the major problem of many diets, which is the elimination of one or more of the essential dietary food groups from meals. The Mediterranean diet includes large portions of fruits, vegetables, bread and other cereals, potatoes, beans, nuts and seeds, small or moderate portions of dairy products (mostly cheese and yogurt), fish and poultry and very little red meat, olive oil as an important monounsaturated fat source, and eggs (less than four times a week). The Mediterranean diet is low in saturated fat, total fat and cholesterol and rich in essential vitamins and minerals including magnesium, potassium and calcium as well as protein and fiber.

What is the Truth About Vitamins?

Vitamins and minerals are substances that your body needs in small quantities in order to function properly. In most cases your body does not make the vitamins and minerals it needs, so they must be consumed on a regular basis. For healthy adults who get a balanced diet, the evidence is split on the benefit of vitamin supplementation. It is felt that anyone who cannot match the recommendations of the new food pyramid should take a daily supplement. Typically anyone

Carlos, Sr.'s O2 for Caregivers

EATING WELL TO STAY FIT

Before Cammy and Blake came back home to South Carolina, I was losing weight. I didn't care for myself physically as I should have, and lacked the motivation to make balanced meals. I wasn't exercising, either, and my health suffered. If this sounds like you, then make sure to:

- Know your body or stay receptive to the insight of someone who does.
- Learn about a balanced diet—and then stick to it.
- Take a multi-vitamin if your doctor agrees.
- Drink lots of water to keep your body hydrated at all times.
- Make the time for regular exercise.

eating fewer than 1600 calories per day, and vegetarians, will have difficulty matching the requirements and should use supplements. Because of their unique needs, all caregivers who are 65 years of age and older should discuss the need for supplements with their health care provider.

What is a Healthy Diet for Seniors?

For most of us, our appetite decreases as we age. A simple explanation is that we use less energy as we age, so the total number of calories we need for daily living also decreases. For example, a woman's caloric intake decreases, on average, from 2,200 calories a day at age 25 to 1,800 calories a day by age 75. But it is critical to understand that, despite the changes in our appetites over time, the nutritional needs of the body do not decrease: we still need the same proteins, carbohydrates, vitamins and minerals that we have always needed.

Lower calorie intake means that elderly consumers must make every calorie count in order to get enough of the essential nutrients needed for healthy living. The "70+ Food Pyramid"developed by researchers at Tufts University outlines the "nutrient dense" choices for seniors in each food category, emphasizing whole grain foods, varied colored fruits and vegetables, low-fat dairy products and lean meats, fish and poultry. More about the 70+ Food Pyramid can be found on www.nutrition.tufts.edu/pyramid.

Update *Your* Food Pyramid

Almost anyone looking over these food guidelines would have lots of ways to make improvements in their diets. But changing what you are used to eating is a challenge, and like all challenges it can seem daunting to get started. But now you've educated yourself and are armed with new facts about a proper diet. You are ready to take action. Start with Step 1 and don't look back!

Step 1: Go to your doctor for a complete physical examination. Find out what your ideal weight should be. Discuss whether any medical condition you may have or the medications you are taking will limit the dietary adjustments you are planning.

Step 2: Get a personal nutrition and diet update. You can do it yourself by following the guidelines found at http://www.mypyramid.gov or you can get a professional dietician or nutritionist to help you. At least three times a week, take some time to think about a healthy and nutritious diet. Once you get into the habit of thinking about what you eat, you will find it much easier to stick with a proper diet.

Step 3: Start planning meals. The same website noted above has an interactive meal planning program called My Pyramid Menu Planner that will lead you through the steps to create a meal plan one week at a time. You can start with just one meal at a time. Extensive sample menus are available to get you started. If you do not use the internet, ask your personal physician to print out the materials for you. Your public library would likely do the same.

Nutrition and Weight Loss - The Payoff

"Daddy certainly doesn't make fun of my 'California cooking' anymore, well, not much anyway!" Cammy says. "Making healthy meals for him made us all more aware of our diets, and we're all reaping the benefits, even now."

You may have noticed that there has been very little discussion to this point about weight loss or weight gain. This is because if you follow these nutritional guidelines, your weight will usually fall in line all by itself. Remember however, that to achieve proper nutrition, you must exercise as well as consume the proper quantities of the right food. Putting the two together is the only way to achieve a healthy nutritional balance.

Nutritional balance is vital for the caregiver. It sets the stage for increased physical energy and should increase the comfort you feel about your body as you age. Sound nutrition and diet leading to ideal weight decrease the likelihood of developing diabetes, hypertension, or worsening those illnesses if you have them. Good nutrition will increase your emotional energy and increase the quality of interactions with your loved ones.

CHAPTER 6

Brain Fitness and Sleep

*C*arlos Jr.: *For most of the last twenty years, the Gibbons family and the Richardson family have celebrated summer by taking week- long beach vacations together. I'd get up early in the morning before the others. Since I didn't want to make noise and wake anyone, I didn't turn on a T.V. Instead, I'd go grab the paper and start doing the crossword puzzle. When we got back to Columbia, I just kept on doing them. So now I'm a regular visitor to Columbia's "The State" newspaper's crossword. It's about 20 minutes of mental exercise that I enjoy. I don't put any pressure on myself. There are times when I can't finish and sometimes I don't get to it until the evening. I think it's helped me retain the title of local "trivia king," at least as far as my family is concerned.*

I have always been a trivia buff and I do tend to absorb and remember a lot of useless information. But the ability has stood me in good stead for Trivial Pursuit nights at a few of the local pubs. I guess trivia is in the Gibbons family genes, since my daughter Kelly is a big "Jeopardy" fan. She and I watch it together. Most of the time we are wrong, but it's a good time.

I don't want to sound like I am making light of the importance of keeping mentally sharp throughout one's life, particularly because of what the family has gone through with Mom. I do worry about my memory. Being a lawyer, I need to have command of a set of facts at a moment's notice. It would put me out of business if I lost my memory. But that was not my main motivation. Remember, I started the puzzles way back when, before all of this started with Grandma and then Mom. With it being in the family, I'd be less than candid to say that that the possibility of memory loss doesn't cross my mind. But I don't obsess about it.

I think staying engaged in life is the key to staying sharp. I'm staying employed, not retiring. And besides, lawyers around here don't retire; they just work till they drop. Most of my older colleagues, if they have the ability to keep working, do. And they sure seem to enjoy it. Law is good for that. I have a friend whose dad is 85 and still working. Another gentleman nearby is north of 85 and still does trial work. And he'll whip your behind in court! There are plenty of examples in town. Now, I don't say I want to be one of them working at 85, but I'd love to have the mental ability at that age to keep working.

As more families like the Gibbon's tackle the long term challenges of caregiving, the benefits of brain fitness are becoming more and more evident. It is now recognized that staying mentally active, beginning in adolescence and continuing through adulthood, lowers the rate of memory decline and improves the quality of the way we think. This quality, known as brain fitness, refers to how well our brains take in and process information from various sources, the way in which we use our cognitive processes to evaluate that information, and how we respond to the information that has been processed. A simple example is seeing a red light (the information we receive), recognizing that a red light means "stop" (understanding the need for action) and knowing when and how to apply the brake (responding appropriately to the information processed).

Brain fitness is valuable for other reasons, too. First, the thinking we do on a day to day basis, both consciously and unconsciously, helps keep our bodies functioning well. An example is eating and drinking. The natural signals our bodies send us in response to hunger and thirst allow us to know when we need to eat and drink without taking time to think about it. Second, brain fitness allows us to feel confident about making decisions—both the mundane decisions and the more challenging ones that caregivers must face. Ultimately, maintaining a high level of brain fitness allows us to live well and maintain our independence throughout our lives.

How the Brain Ages

In some respects, the brain continues to function as it always has regardless of how old you are. You can expect that abilities known as *preserved functions* to remain sharp for your entire life. Preserved functions include:

- Attention span: watching a television program, reading a book
- Remote memory: remembering your wedding day.
- Everyday communication skills: social greetings, telephone etiquette.
- Visual perception: the ability to understand what is being seen.
- Knowledge of syntax: understanding written and spoken language.

Some functions in every brain are affected by age. Known as *declining functions*, these are the annoying glitches in memory, attention and ability that we all know as "senior moments." Examples of these include the following:

- Speed of processing memories: "Oh here he comes...

What's his name?" Later at dinner: "It's George, of course!"

- Fluency: coming to a dead stop in the middle of a sentence and searching for a word.
- Naming objects: "Honey, can you find the ...the.... 'thing'?" (the remote control, the keys, etc.).
- Cognitive flexibility: difficulty learning how to work the new DVD player, cell phone, etc.
- Complex visuospatial skills: difficulty judging available turning time while driving.
- Complex logical analysis: following multi-step processes, such as balancing a checkbook.
- Selective attention: multi-tasking becomes more difficult.

Is it Normal Aging or a Memory Loss Disorder?

As we get older, we all dread "senior moments." What we all want to know is, are these momentary lapses in memory just normal aging or are they a sign of something more serious? The answer is, it all depends.

First, it is vital to understand that Alzheimer's disease is a *disease*. It is vastly different from having a normal 80 year-old brain that may take longer to retrieve the name of an acquaintance from its memory bank, a phenomenon known as *age-related memory loss or decline*. These transient memory lapses are not the same as losing the ability to make memories; they are instead an indication of a slowing ability to retrieve memories. One of the first symptoms of the presence of Alzheimer's disease is often memory loss. However, to truly be Alzheimer's disease and not just age-related decline, there must be an indication of a decline in more than just memory retrieval. Examples include the loss of an understanding of the date and time or a loss of language abilities. The changes must progress over time and they must impair one's ability to function on a day to day basis. If you or your loved one is concerned that what is being experienced is something more than merely a normal slowing down of abilities, take your concerns to your doctor as soon as possible.

Caregivers and the "Senior Moment Syndrome"

Caregivers must be as intellectually alert as possible, particularly when called upon to make decisions for the person in need. But the stress and anxiety, together with the poor eating habits and disruptions in sleep that can come with caring for a loved one, can cause a decline in brain fitness. In some cases, inattention or distraction can make it difficult to think clearly. Here is an example: The phone rings. It's the adult day care center changing the time of the caregivers' pot luck dinner to 6 P.M. from 5 P.M. During the conversation, your loved one calls from the other room for help getting a book down from a high shelf. At the same time, the kitchen timer goes off, telling you the casserole is ready. You hang up the phone and help your loved one retrieve the book, and while doing so you realize your loved one needs to change (again) for dinner. Unfortunately, you forget about the casserole until it's too late! Combine these day to day factors with other illnesses that can affect memory and thinking and it becomes clear why caregivers are at increased risk for problems with thinking and memory that are known as the "senior moment syndrome." While it does not usually signify future disease, it can be extremely frustrating, especially as you are trying to keep straight the details and demands of your loved one's care. So how do you combat "senior moment syndrome"? A brain fitness routine is a good start.

NORMAL AGING-RELATED MEMORY CHANGES

- Forgetting names and appointments.
- Occasionally forgetting why you entered a room.
- Occasional sad or blue days.
- Sometimes having trouble finding the right word.
- Forgetting the date or the day of the week, or where you were going.
- Making a questionable decision from time to time.
- Temporarily misplacing your keys or wallet.
- Mild personality changes
- Feeling weary of work or social obligations.

SYMPTOMS OF ALZHEIMER'S DISEASE

- Forgetting recently learned information.
- Difficulty performing job-related tasks that had been well performed in the past.
- Loss of initiative.
- Unusual mood swings.
- Changes in personality.
- Difficulty performing common tasks, such as preparing a meal.
- Forgetting simple words and/or substituting unusual words.
- Getting lost in familiar surroundings.
- Poor or decreased judgment.
- Difficulty with complex tasks.
- Misplacing items and putting them in unusual locations (not just forgetting where your wallet is, but putting your wallet in the refrigerator and not thinking it's too unusual when it's found there).

Does Brain Exercise Work?

Taylor: My grandma and my great grandma stayed home with their kids. Don't get me wrong; I know that can be very challenging! But they didn't get much real "brain exercise" like you'd get in academic or workplace areas. Sometimes I wonder if that contributed to their getting Alzheimer's, or if it made the disease worse. It's made me think about balancing a career and family so that I can lower my own risk.

There is good evidence that brain exercise is helpful. Some of the forgetfulness and loss of mental acuity that come with aging are caused, at least in part, by non-use. Seniors engaged in mentally stimulating activities have been shown to have lower rates of developing dementia. In 2003, researchers found that among leisure activities, reading, playing board games, playing musical instruments, and dancing were associated with a reduced risk of dementia.[2]

Just as a program for physical fitness includes a variety of exercises, brain fitness is most successful if you pay attention to the right mix of exercises that help the brain stay fit and functional. As you think about planning your own brain fitness program, consider these four key factors:

RELAX

Relaxation has been shown to help keep thinking clear in older adults, as it does in people of all ages. One way to relax is through meditation, which works to lower stress levels and which leads to

---

2 J. Verghese, R. Lipton, M. Katz, C. Hall, C. Drby, G. Kuslansky, A. Ambrose, M. Sliwinski, H. Buschle. *Leisure Activities and the Risk of Dementia in the Elderly,* New England Journal of Medicine; 2003; 348:2508-16

TEN TIPS FOR BETTER BRAIN FITNESS

1. Learn what the "It" is in "Use It or Lose It". A basic understanding of how the brain works will serve you well to appreciate your brain as a living and constantly-developing organ with billions of neurons and synapses (see Chapter 2).

2. Take care of your nutrition. The brain consists of only 2% of total body mass but consumes over 20% of the nutrients and oxygen we take in. As a general rule, you don't need expensive nutritional supplements; just make sure you eat healthy foods (see Chapter 5).

3. Keep Moving. Remember the brain is part of the body. Things that exercise the body can also help sharpen your brain: Physical exercise improves circulation and overall health of the neurons involved in making memories and thinking (See Chapter 9).

4. Be positive. Look forward to every day in a constructive way. Stress and anxiety, whether created by external events or by your own thoughts, actually kill neurons and prevents the creation of new ones.

5. Thrive on Learning and Mental Challenges. It's never too late to learn something new. The best workout for the brain is to learn and adapt to new challenges.

6. Relax. Let your mind work, stress-free.

7. Explore. Adapting to new locations forces you to pay more attention to your environment.

8. Get some sleep! Get enough sleep overnight and take and nap during the day if you need it to recharge your batteries.

9. Friends forever. We are "social animals" and need social interaction (see Chapter 10).

10. Laugh. Often. Especially to cognitively complex humor, full of twists and surprises.

better brain function even as your days get more stressful. Daily prayer or journaling can also be effective.

GET MOVING

Physical activity can help keep your brain working in top form. Part of the benefit comes from improved blood circulation that encourages the growth of new brain cells by increasing oxygen flow to your brain. That same circulation boosts other growth factors, such as what is known as *brain-derived neurotrophic factor*, which helps new nerve cells to survive. Finally, it is believed that exercise increases the levels of some of the neurotransmitters in your brain that play a role in thinking. Refer to Chapter 4 of this book for exercise tips.

DON'T RETIRE FROM LIFE

Do you know what the definition of "retire" is? "To withdraw, or go away or apart, to a place of privacy, shelter, or seclusion." Don't do it! Or if you do retire, don't put down your intellect and pick up the remote. Researchers have found that that cognitively active seniors were 2.6 times less likely to develop dementia than those who were less active intellectually.[3] Even with the pressures and time demands of caregiving, you need to find time to stay engaged with the outside world. Learning new things, such as playing a musical instrument or a foreign language, is a very effective way of keeping your mind intellectually fit.

---

3 Wilson, R.S, Scherr, P.A., Schneider, J.A., Tang, A., Bennett, D.A., *Relation of Cognitive Activity to Developing Alzheimer's Disease.* Neurology, 2007 Nov 13: 69 (20):1911-20.Epub 2007 Jun 27.

SOCIALIZE

The well known saying "united we stand, divided we fall" is never more true than when it's applied to caregivers. Social isolation is a common occurrence among caregivers, given the time that is required to give proper care to a loved one. Going to the corner store can become a major undertaking. Dining out with friends becomes difficult as the behaviors of your loved one become unpredictable. Often, the response to these circumstances is to stay home. Resist the urge to cancel your plans to attend the support group. Don't rely on the neighbor to pick up the few things you need at the store. In each instance, your interaction with the world around you diminishes. While these changes may seem minor, the loss of social activities can be dangerous to your health, since medical research has shown that the more social activities a caregiver is involved with, the less likely she is to have the symptoms of depression.[4] And, as we discussed earlier, depression makes it difficult to think clearly and efficiently and contributes to "senior moment syndrome".

Brain Fitness - The Payoff

For the weary and worried caregiver, the "10 Minutes A Day" brain fitness plan (see next box) will help you feel stronger with each passing day, even as your caregiving challenges become more and more complex and taxing. Over time, your brain fitness program will help you feel more confident making decisions, managing day to day care issues, and making long range plans. You will also reap personal dividends as you pay more attention to your overall health and

---

4 Schulz, R. Beach., *SR Caregiving as a Risk Factor for Mortality: The Caregiver Effects Study.Journal of the America Medical Association*, 1999;282 (23): 2215-2219.

10 MINUTES A DAY FOR BRAIN FITNESS

If you can find just 10 minutes a day, you can improve your brain fitness! Each day choose ONE of these activities from the 4 major areas that will help improve your brain fitness.

Relaxation
- Meditation
- Journal
- Prayer or Bible reading

Physical activity
- Caregiver Exercise Circuit (see Chapter 4)
- Walk around the house or block
- 10 minutes of Sit and Be Fit (a PBS program, check your local listings)

Brain Activity
- Do the daily crossword or word jumble
- Put 25 more pieces into a jigsaw puzzle
- Write a poem
- Learn five more words of another language
- Learn a new song on the keyboard or other musical instrument

Social activity
- Call a shut-in caregiver or relative
- Invite a neighbor over for coffee and a chat
- Answer emails

fitness and to your cognitive and emotional stability. You will increase the quality of interactions with your loved ones and increase the comfort you feel about yourself and your role as caregiver.

Sleep is Good—When You Can Get It

Carlos, Sr.: Before Jean went to live in the facility, for almost two years we had ladies that came in to help out. We had one lady Monday through Thursday and another from Friday through Sunday. But I would still have her at night by myself. She would fall asleep O.K. but then she'd get up in the middle of the night and just roam around. Then she would not go back to bed. I would have to stay up with her the whole time. She'd go from room to room, opening and closing a chest of drawers, or putting things into and taking them out of her pocketbook, or smoking cigarettes. There was no sleep involved after that. Many times I'd be afraid she would set the house on fire with a cigarette..

Later, after Jean moved to the nursing home, the nighttime was difficult for me for other reasons. I think it was just not having anyone there after 47 years of marriage. Being there by myself, before Cammy and Blake came, that was tough. I was more tired. I went to bed earlier. But even though I went to bed early, I only slept during the first part of the night. Sometimes there would be things on my mind. Sometimes that's when I'd write a poem. But after a while, the tiredness made even that difficult.

Everyone loves to sleep. But sleep is more than just a relaxing activity. Our bodies *need* to rest each day to restore and grow, leaving us refreshed and ready for the next day. When sleep is interrupted we feel it right away. Miss one day of sleep and mental processes become less efficient and your mood in general can become depressed. For caregivers, issues such as the uncertainty of the future, the difficulty in finding help and the inability to understand options for treatment all add up to a great deal of anxiety during the day. At night, when it's time for the body and mind to calmly drift into sleep, these issues can create a number of different sleep-related problems. Chronic sleep deprivation robs us of our emotional and physical well being and in turn limits our ability to interact well with our loved one.

Insomnia

In general, insomnia is the inability to fall asleep or to remain asleep through the night. The most common forms of insomnia are when a person can't fall asleep at the beginning of the night or it takes a long time (more than 30 to 45 minutes) to fall asleep. It can come after a sleep interruption, where a person wakes up many times each night and cannot fall back to sleep easily. Others find waking up early and being unable to get back to sleep is the major problem. Finally, there are those who have a general sense of waking up feeling tired and remaining that way during most days. All of these forms of insomnia can be caused by many things, including emotionally charged circumstances such as losing a loved one or lifestyle issues such as drinking alcohol or caffeine.

What Causes Insomnia?

Insomnia can be caused by a number of factors, and sometimes by a combination of them. Among caregivers, it's very common for insomnia to be brought on by stress, since anxiety over day to day or long-term concerns may keep a caregiver's mind too alert, preventing sleep. Depression can also be a factor, as it can cause chemical changes in the brain that may affect sleeping habits. Medications can cause insomnia, too. Many over-the-counter medications, including some decongestants and weight-loss products, contain caffeine and other stimulants. Antihistamines like benadryl may initially cause grogginess which can promote falling asleep, but they can worsen urinary problems, causing sleep interruptions. They're especially hard on older adults and can lead to confusion as well. Medical conditions such as *gastroesophageal reflux disease* (hearburn), arthritis, sleep apnea and restless leg syndrome (RLS) can also play a part in causing insomnia. If you have been having symptoms for one month or longer, or you feel the need to take an over-the-counter medication to help you get to sleep, you should speak first to your doctor. He or she can review the long list of possible causes and recommend treatment options.

Sleep and the Older Caregiver

As we get older it can be more difficult to get a good night's rest, even though the total sleep we need stays about the same. Older adults experience changes in the sleep cycle that impact nighttime routines. For example, more time is spent in lighter stages of sleep than in the deep stages of sleep, called *Non-REM sleep*, which is the time during the sleep cycle when restorative sleep occurs. Because you're sleeping more lightly, you're also more likely to wake up due to physical discomfort, such as having to go to the bathroom or an aching back. Another consequence of aging is that your internal clock, the natural signal your body gives you to let you know it is time to sleep, tends to "advance" so that you are tired earlier in the evening and consequently wake up earlier in the morning.

TIPS FOR GOOD NIGHT'S REST

- Follow a regular schedule: go to sleep and wake up at the same time.
- Do not nap during the day (this is only true if you are having trouble sleeping at night. Otherwise, new evidence suggests a nap in the early afternoon can be beneficial).
- Get natural light in the afternoon each day.
- Be careful about what you eat. Don't drink beverages with caffeine late in the day.
- Don't drink alcohol or smoke. Even small amounts of alcohol make it harder to stay asleep and the nicotine in cigarettes is a stimulant.
- Exercise at regular times each day. Try to finish your workout at least three hours before bedtime.
- Create a comfortable place to sleep. The room should be dark, well ventilated, and quiet.
- Develop a bedtime routine. Do the same things each night to tell your body it is time to wind down.
- Use the 10 minute limit: It's a good idea never to stay in bed for more than 10 minutes if you cannot fall asleep. Don't toss and turn. Get out of bed and do something relaxing then try again.
- Save the bed for sleep and sex only, not for reading, watching TV, or other activities.

In addition to these physiological changes, there are other changes that can impact sleep in older caregivers. As an older caregiver, you may not be able to participate in the leisure sports or fitness activities you used to, and physical activity helps promote a good night's sleep. In other cases, a health condition can disrupt sleep. The chronic pain of conditions such as arthritis or back problems as well as depression, anxiety and stress can all interfere with sleep. Older men often develop an enlargement of the prostate gland (*benign prostatic hyperplasia*), which can cause the need to urinate frequently, interrupting sleep. In women, hot flashes that accompany menopause can be equally disruptive.

Discovering the Problem

To get to the bottom of what is causing your sleep disturbance, a good place to start is with a *sleep diary*. Keeping track of the details of how you sleep, such as the time you are going to sleep, what seems to interrupt your sleep, and how much you are sleeping dur-

A Typical Sleep Diary

DAY	Bed Time	Woke Up	Reason	Activity
Monday	10 P.M.	1 A.M.	Not sure	Read in bed
Tuesday	10:30 P.M.	3 A.M.	Bathroom	Bathoom and Bed
Wednesday	3 A.M.	Still awake	Unknown	Trying to sleep
Thursday	10 P.M.	Slept all night		

WHEN YOUR LOVED ONE IS KEEPING YOU AWAKE

Often, your sleep is interrupted by your loved one who, in the case of Alzheimer's disease, can be up in the middle of the night, dressed and ready to begin his work day. If this happens to you, make a note to yourself that includes the date, time, and any pertinent factors about the awakening. If this behavior becomes a pattern and happens more than three times a week, you should speak with your loved one's physician to find out the reasons for his behavior and try to find a solution.

In most instances, the best way to correct this problem is to "redirect, don't reorient." Trying to convince your loved one that he does not have to go to work is not likely to be effective. Instead, go along with his plan, but mention the late start that day due to a staff meeting or that the shop is closed for the weekend.

Redirect your loved one to some "at-the-ready" activities you know will distract him from the idea that he must be up and about. Ideally, use relaxing activities that are conducive to getting your loved one back to bed, such as listening to soft music in a rocking chair or looking over a photo album. Don't insist on changing clothes again unless it seems to help move your loved one back to sleeping.

ing the day can help you identify patterns that may be causing your sleep trouble. Your physician may be able to look over the diary and think about medications or factors related to your medical history that might be causing your problem.

As you are waiting to talk with your doctor, be careful about choosing an over the counter medication. Older caregivers should be wary of the "P.M." types of preparations, since the active ingredient, benadryl, produces side effects that include confusion and urinary retention. *All* prescription sleep aids induce gait instability because of drowsiness. For older adults who need to use the bathroom at night, this can increase the risk of falling. For all ages, there is a potential for dependency on the medication as well as continued drowsiness during the day, which may impair driving or other skilled mental and physical activities.

A Good Night's Sleep - The Payoff

As a well rested, physically fit caregiver, you are stronger and more effective. Your emotional stability brings greater peace and well being to your family. Your loved one can sense the gentler environment and becomes less tense. Not only are you able to provide better care, but your body is functioning more easily and with greater energy. This is a perfect example of how the Three E's are directly relate to each other. You have built from a base of Education, Empowering yourself towards more Energy. You feel your "zest for life" returning. Your brain is firing faster and is able to handle the many decisions and demands required of you a little more easily.

But before your mind is free to become more energized, you may have to get through some of the emotional hurdles that can complicate your days as a caregiver. In the next chapters we'll examine how emotional problems may be holding you back on your road to a rewarding life, and how to step beyond them and free yourself and your energy for growth and happiness.

PART III:

CARING FOR THE CAREGIVER'S MIND

Tis the mind makes the body rich.

—Shakespeare

CHAPTER 7

Coping with Depression and Anxiety

Depression

*L*eeza: *Bad news has no regard for timing. Your bubble of domestic bliss is not immune, nor is your job or career. I was happily mothering my children and producing and hosting my own talk show on Paramount's Stage 26 when Mom's stage went dark. My anxiety spread to every aspect of my life and as much as I tried to present a facade of calm and acceptance, my persona never lasted past my driveway and once home, I became as tightly wound up as an angry fist. I snapped at the kids, withdrew from my husband and stayed up until dawn searching and searching for the latest treatments, the slimmest hope.*

As Mom declined, I was trapped on a tilt-a-whirl of emotion. I managed to convince myself that if I just did more, she would be O.K. The talk show ended its run and I immediately went on to the next stop on my career train, hosting the nightly entertainment news magazine Extra. I was all coifed and poised in front of the camera as I delivered the latest celebrity headlines, but the minute the lights went out on the stage, I fell apart. I spent most afternoons leaving through the back door of the lot to wander the neighborhood streets trying to reclaim some control over myself. But bad news can't be controlled and I realized that I was no match for its increasing shadow over my life. My marriage was strained to the breaking point and I was depressed. I needed to let go of the way things were and accept this beast which had pulled up a chair to my dinner table.

I sought the help of a therapist. It turned out to be more than a lifeline, it was the exploration I needed to reclaim my sanity. Robert, my therapist, provided a safe sanctuary in which to share my feelings. Jamie Huysman, the co-author of this book, was my tether to what would become a new life and a new sense of purpose. He was the friend who always had time for me, who never judged and who always reminded me to be kind to myself. When I was unsure, he was certain. When I was a squishy ball of frayed nerves, he was solid, strong and firm in his belief that I could make a difference. Jamie showed me how to fulfill the promise I made to my mother, to tell her story so that others might be helped and inspired.

Leeza found out the hard way that no amount of family or career distractions could save her from the tidal wave of emotions that can arise when one is taking care of a loved one with a memory loss disorder. She became trapped in a seemingly endless cycle of grief.

Grief is healthy when it helps us to cope with painful changes in our lives, allowing us to heal from loss and embrace a new reality. Healthy grief releases feelings rather than keeping them bottled up inside and lets us move forward in life with renewed vitality. The ideal result of grief is achieving *closure*, or an end to our feelings of loss or pain. However, when closure is not reached within a reasonable amount of time, normal grief can become depression, and depression came close to consuming Leeza's spirit.

Coping with a loved one's dementia demands a great deal from caregivers, who often struggle to make do without a strong support system in place to help shoulder the burden. Caregivers are forced

Carlos, Sr.'s O2 for Caregivers

FIGHTING GRIEF

When I finally lost Jean, I lost not only a loved one; I lost my fulltime "job" of caregiving. Combined, it was a huge void into which terrible grief could have entered. When your loved one passes, don't waste any time slipping into depression! I found as many things as possible to engage my mind and keep myself busy. Try these:

- Join a support group
- Find a therapist who understands caregiving and the complicated grief it brings
- Return to the hobbies and social activities that once interested you.
- Join an organization like Leeza's Place to volunteer and give back.
- Take the time to honor all the sacred memories through journaling, poetry or scrapbooking.

to let go of a loved one little by little, again and again, sometimes over a span of many years, and grief over these losses is often experienced over and over. The grief associated with caregiving is uniquely burdensome: often, when illness and subsequent death strike, a caregiver must face not only the loss of the loved one, but loss of control and loss of independence, as well as the possible loss of his job and plans for the future. This experience may explain why caregivers are more likely to suffer from symptoms of depression: a recent study of the emotional state of caregivers reports that up to 60% are, to some degree, depressed.

While feelings of sadness associated with grief lessen with time, depression can dim the joy of life for months, even years. People who have experienced depression are familiar with its disabling

THERAPY OPTIONS FOR TREATING DEPRESSION:

- How we can change what we do (Behavioral therapy) .
- Changing how think about things (Cognitive therapy).
- Exploring how we relate to others (Interpersonal therapy).
- Finding solutions to present and future problems (Solution- Focused therapy).

The decision about which kind of therapy is best for you should be made in consultation with your doctor.

heaviness, which is markedly different from normal sadness. Depressive illness is not just about "having the blues" for too long. It interferes with daily life and causes pain and suffering not only for those who have the disorder, but for those around them.

"I was heartbroken and stunned when we first heard Art's diagnosis", recalls Rose, one of our Leeza's Place clients, whose husband was diagnosed with Alzheimer's disease. "It was so hard to accept that he was really ill. Eventually though, I moved into my new role and our new relationship and made the best of it. Then suddenly, after 42 years of marriage, Art didn't know who I was." At this point, Rose experienced what she called "a loss of meaning", not just in her role as caregiver, but in her life. She stopped visiting with friends and called her children less and less often. "I couldn't bring myself to leave the house much. I had been taking Art to church with me every week, but I stopped taking him anywhere and we ended up at home in front of the T.V. most of the time. I found myself crying the first thing in the morning most days, or wanting to stay in bed all day. Finally my daughter came to visit and convinced me to talk to my doctor about what I was feeling."

Like Leeza, Rose was lucky to have someone who could see what was happening and encourage her to seek professional help. Although she had been able to experience healthy grief at the onset of the disease, Rose began to experience depression once her husband lost his memory of her.

While grieving, you might be fairly dysfunctional for a short period of time, unwilling to do the things you might normally do. However, a person experiencing healthy grief recognizes that life does go on and eventually seeks to move forward, with energy and healing. *Clinical depression*, on the other hand, lasts without relief. It sinks into you and prevents you from moving forward in life. You might instead obsess about the perceived futility of life and not even take comfort from talking with others. Depression may isolate you entirely, and in isolation the depression only deepens. You may feel exhausted, worthless, helpless and hopeless, negative views that typically do not accurately reflect the actual circumstances of your life.

The danger of depression is physical as well as mental. Caregivers who suffer from depression tend to have weakened immune systems and an increased chance of developing chronic illness. Depression can increase the risk of osteoporosis and high blood pressure and also increase levels of *stress hormones*, such as adrenaline and cortisol, which can, over the long run, increase the risk of heart disease and digestive problems. It can even shrink the hippocampus, the area of the brain involved with learning and memory. Because of the toll depression takes on caregivers and on those around them, it is important to recognize the warning signs of depression and understand how they differ from necessary and healthy grieving.

Recognizing Depression

Depression must first be recognized before it can be treated. But many don't realize the need for help because they assume that it is only natural to be feeling sad, given the stresses and sorrow caused by a loved one's memory loss. If you are concerned about the possibility of suffering from depression, look at the following list. If you have five or more of the symptoms listed and they have lasted for two weeks or more, you may be at risk for depression:

- Sadness most of the day.
- A markedly diminished interest or pleasure in activities.
- Significant weight loss or weight gain, or a decrease or increase in appetite.
- Insomnia or *hypersomnia*, prolonged nighttime sleeping

or daytime sleepiness.
- *Psychomotor agitation* which includes excessive pacing, handwringing, or nail biting.
- Fatigue or loss of energy.
- Feelings of worthlessness or excessive or inappropriate feelings of guilt.
- A diminished ability to think or concentrate or indecisiveness.
- Recurring thoughts of death (not just fear of dying), or recurring thoughts of suicide.

Treating Depression

People with depression cannot simply "snap out of it" and feel better spontaneously, nor is recovery from clinical depression a matter of will-power. However, the disease is highly treatable with competent care.

Finding help requires seeking help; your doctor is an invaluable resource when it comes to obtaining effective treatment. Unfortunately, many times a doctor will miss the signs of depression in caregivers. Being a caregiver is a red flag for depression, yet only a third of all physicians inquire of their caregiver patients about depression. It's easier, after all, to limit an examination to questions about blood pressure or diabetes. Caregivers need to be proactive about depression; they must bring up concerns or questions about it with their doctors, otherwise, unexpressed feelings and concerns, accompanied by a sense of isolation, can worsen depression, creating a vicious cycle of increasing isolation and pain.

Caregivers who are clinically depressed often think that they just "need a break" and take a short time off from their duties. But often they return to find themselves in the same situation that caused the depression in the first place. In order to truly overcome clinical depression, psychological issues must be dealt with, generally through counseling.

Depression can result in chemical imbalances in the brain which can be addressed with medications called *antidepressants*. In many cases, these medications can help a person fell better but do not eliminate the cause of the depression. Thus, like aspirin, antidepressants can reduce symptoms while leaving the cause of the pain untreated. For example, antidepressants can lift the dark, heavy moods of depression, but a caregiver will still need to address the difficulties at home in order to recover thoroughly. The degree of improvement, from a little relief from the symptoms to complete remission, depends on a variety of factors related to the individual

THE UNITED STATES FOOD AND DRUG ADMINISTRATION (F.D.A.) RECOMMENDS THAT YOU ASK YOUR DOCTOR THE FOLLOWING QUESTIONS ABOUT ANY DRUGS THAT ARE PRESCRIBED:

- What is the name of the medication, and what is it supposed to do?
- How and when do I take it, and when do I stop taking it?
- What foods, drinks, other medications, or activities should I avoid while taking the prescribed medication?
- What are the side effects, and what should I do if they occur?
- Is there any written information available about the medication?

and the severity of the depression being treated.

The length of time one continues with antidepressant medication treatment is largely determined by the individual and her level of depression, rather than the situation that may have triggered the disease. Typically, a doctor will prescribe medications for six to twelve months and then stop the treatment to see how a person responds. Frequently, some resolution has occurred in this time and further treatment is unnecessary. Many depressed people need medication just for a single period such as this, and then never have to take it again. For some depressions however, medication may have to be taken intermittently or perhaps indefinitely. Like any medication, antidepressants do not produce the same effect in everyone. Some people may respond better to one medication than another. Some may need larger dosages than others. Some experience annoying side effects, while others do not. Age, sex, body size, body chemistry, physical illnesses and their treatments, diet, and habits such as smoking, are some of the factors that can influence a medication's effects. Sometimes it takes several attempts to find the types of medication and counseling that work best, and it is essential to work with your doctor to find effective treatment.

Physicians will recommend a particular antidepressant based on the symptoms that are present. Relief does not come immediately; it usually takes between one and three weeks for change to occur. Some symptoms of depression diminish early in treatment; others take a while longer to respond. For instance, energy level or sleeping and eating patterns may improve before the depressed mood lifts. If there is little or no change in symptoms after five to six weeks, a different medication may be needed. When searching for an effective medication, it is crucial to work closely with your physician and communicate regularly with him or her about any effects, or lack of effects, you might experience.

There are a number of different types of antidepressant medications available. They differ in their side effects and, to some extent, in their level of effectiveness. As we mentioned in Chapter 2, the most commonly prescribed antidepressants are called *selective serotonin reuptake inhibitors* (SSRIs). Some examples of these drugs are fluoxetine (Prozac), fluvoxamine (Luvox), paroxetine (Paxil), and sertraline (Zoloft). Although chemically different from each other, all the SSRI antidepressants act on *serotonin*, a brain neurotransmitter. The F.D.A. has also approved antidepressants that have an effect on serotonin and another neurotransmitter, *norepinephrine*. They are venlafaxine (Effexor) and nefazodone (Serzone). Another of the newer antidepressants, bupropion (Wellbutrin), has more of an effect on norepinephrine and *dopamine*, another brain chemical, than on serotonin and it seems to have fewer side effects than the other types of drugs.

Beyond Depression - The Payoff

When Leeza looks back on her run-in with depression, she is grateful for having been able to get past it. "I realize now that we have to deal with our unhealthy emotions that same as we would any other unhealthy aspect of our being. Beyond depression, there's clarity and strength. There's so much more than just inner happiness and peace: there's peace and happiness that can radiate from you as a gift to others."

What will you be like, freed from depression? Freed from depression, you are better able to adapt to the constant changes in your loved ones' condition and are better equipped to think more realistically about your situations. Without depression, you will be more calm and accepting with your loved one. Without depression, it's easier to see the degenerative disease as a separate entity from your loved one. When your loved one becomes mentally or physically aggressive, as is common, without depression you are more likely to find positive ways to handle the situation, rather than responding in kind and increasing the struggle.

Without depression, you can make better judgments and handle day-to-day tasks more easily and manage future planning with greater clarity and sounder decisions. Without depression, you can pay better attention to your own health and wellness, such as healthy eating and exercise, finding social support, or taking more opportunities for rejuvenation. You can provide greater quality of care to your loved one as well, and studies have shown that a loved one with a strong and healthy caregiver actually manages his own disease better in the long run.

When you are free from depression, you can also find warmth and love in the process of caregiving. Every day provides an opportunity to connect with others, to find some moment of beauty in life, or to be grateful for life itself. Beyond depression, there may still be grief and difficulty, but there is also the possibility of great joy.

Anxiety

Our guest Martha, a sixty three year-old widow, is the caregiver to her sister, who is battling Alzheimer's disease. Several months ago, Martha sold her home in Santa Fe and moved across the country to her sister's place, bringing a few belongings and her old cat, Max. Alhough she loved her job, she had accepted retirement in order to meet her sister's need for constant care. The move went well, and she enjoys the time she has with her sister. She keeps up with the news as often as she can and takes a pottery class once a week, just to "stay alert." All in all, Martha is pretty happy except for her worries about the cat's health. Max became lethargic and sickly when they first arrived at their new home. He quickly recovered but still, Martha worries. She doesn't allow him outside any longer, though Max used to be an outdoor-only cat, and she admits to visiting the veterinarian nearly every week. In fact, she is convinced that the local vet isn't attentive enough and she's been considering hiring someone to watch her sister in order to travel two hours away to a "cat specialist."

Martha isn't crazy, though she feels that way at times. Her obsessive attention to the cat is one way her concern for her sister and her lack of control over her sister's condition manifests itself. After talking with her doctor, Martha realized that she was worrying about more than just Max, for most of the time. In fact, her brain was having trouble "turning off" and she often had trouble sleeping or focusing on one task at a time. Martha had what is called *Generalized Anxiety Disorder.*

WHAT IS ANXIETY?

Unhealthy anxiety is a constant and overwhelming feeling of apprehension, fear, or worry. Most of us have heard of the "fight or flight" response, when our nervous system shifts into high gear in order to deal with danger. This response is literally a life-saver when functioning properly, causing our hearts to pump faster, our breathing to quicken, and our blood pressure to increase in order to make more oxygen available to us so that we can run faster or fight more fiercely. When we experience this in normal life, we are motivated to protect ourselves and our loved ones and can respond faster to threats, such as when a car pulls in front of us suddenly. But when this response gets out of control, our bodies get pummeled by stress hormones and suffer negative consequences.

THE SYMPTOMS OF ANXIETY

Stress kills. Chronic, unchecked stress can lead to such serious conditions as heart attacks and strokes. There is increasing evidence that stress is also a contributing factor to other illness, such as rheumatoid arthritis, diabetes, and frequent colds or respiratory infections. If we are constantly on alert, as we are when anxious, we are depleting our energy stores and compromising our immune systems. Effectively managing one's stress can be a powerful weapon against anxiety and serious illness.

Do you find yourself getting anxious whenever your loved one is out of sight? Are you awake listening for him all night, fearing the worst? Are you up in the middle of the night wondering and fretting about tomorrow, unable to return to sleep? Are you frequently irritable and quick to snap at those around you? Do you jump at sudden noises? Do your thoughts run away with you, making it difficult to stay on task or focus clearly?

It can be difficult to tell if your level of anxiety is too high. A good rule of thumb is to honestly consider how much it impairs your life or keeps you from doing the things you would like to do. Anxiety often becomes a problem after a prolonged period of extreme stress or traumatic change (such as receiving a memory disorder diagnosis). Too much stress and anxiety can seriously affect our ability to focus on coping skills; we feel anxious because we are stressed and we are stressed even more by our anxiety.

Unless we know how to manage anxiety, it can become a chronic condition. Take a look at the following list and see if any of these symptoms apply to you:

- Palpitations.
- Sweating.

- Trembling.
- Shortness of breath.
- A sense of choking.
- Chest pain.
- Dizziness.
- Feeling detached.
- A fear of dying.
- Numbness or tingling.
- Chills or hot flushes.
- Nausea.

If you frequently experience three of more of these symptoms for six months or more at a time, you may have an anxiety disorder. Sometimes, like Martha, we are unaware of our anxiety, but we usually know we feel fatigued or nervous more often than we'd like to feel. Anxiety, like any psychological disorder, is simply a signal that there is something out of balance that needs our attention.

TREATING ANXIETY

Treatments used to help resolve anxiety issues include medications, *cognitive-behavioral therapy*, lifestyle changes, and stress management techniques. But no matter how we approach our healing, we must commit to it in order to transform our anxious, fear-ridden experience into one of greater peace, strength, and energy.

Medication

Most anxiety disorders are not solely psychological, but also have a biological component that often responds to medications which help repair mood-affecting chemical imbalances in the brain. The benefits of these medications appear to be limited to the time when they are actively being taken, so for this reason, medications are often prescribed for just a short period of time, to ease the immediate symptoms of anxiety and facilitate counseling.

Therapy

Most patients with anxiety disorders will be best treated with *cognitive-behavioral therapy,* often in combination with medication. Cognitive-behavioral therapy works on the principle that our thoughts influence the way we feel and behave. In other words, an anxious person interprets certain situations as dangerous, causing anxiety symptoms and a desire to escape. For example, when our loved one becomes verbally aggressive, we might think, "I'm a terrible caregiver; of course he's sick of me." This thought leads us to feel badly about ourselves and our situations and creates anxiety. We would have a very different reaction to the same event if we thought instead, "This is the disease talking. I know I am doing the best I can." Cognitive behavioral therapy teaches you to change the way you think in order to change how you feel. This does not mean that it is "all in your head" but rather means that you can learn new sets of skills and techniques to gain more control over your feelings and how you react in various situations.

Lifestyle Changes

Simple lifestyle changes can help us to recover from anxiety. As we discussed in Chapter 4, exercise is a powerful tool that can be used to overcome both anxiety and depression and offers many other benefits as well. A healthy diet, along with exercise, promotes optimal brain health, which directly impacts our emotional well being.

Cutting down on substances such as caffeine and alcohol is a sure way to turn the odds in our favor.

Stress Management Techniques

It is important throughout the caregiving journey to monitor our stress levels. When we are overwhelmed but tempted to just "deal with it", without taking concrete steps to reduce our stress, it negatively affects those we care for as well as ourselves. The symptoms of anxiety are the body's way of letting us know it needs to relax. When our bodies are relaxed, we can cope better with our lives. Learn to deal with stress by practicing the techniques which can relax your body and mind regardless of external events. In addition to getting enough rest and relaxation, exercising and following a healthy diet, techniques such as *imagery, meditation,* and *progressive muscular relaxation* are effective tools for relieving stress.

Imagery is a potent method of stress reduction, especially when combined with physical relaxation methods such as deep breathing. The idea behind the use of imagery is that you can create a very relaxing situation in your mind, which will settle your anxiety and help you calm yourself. The more intensely you imagine the situa-

> **Try It:** Imagine a scene, place or event that you remember as safe, peaceful, restful, beautiful and happy. You can bring all your senses into the image with, for example, sounds of running water and birds, the smell of cut grass, the taste of a favorite food, the warmth of the sun, and so on. Use the imagined place as a retreat from stress and pressure.

tion, the more relaxing the experience will be.

Meditation is a useful and practical technique for managing stress, with strong psychological *and* physical benefits. It can help rest your body, allow stress hormones to subside, and occupy your mind so that unpleasant, stressful thoughts do not intrude. There are many forms of meditation, all of which can be learned on your own and practiced almost anywhere. The actual practice can range from sustaining one thought to simply paying attention to our thought habits. One of the most common forms of meditation is breath practice, which involve sitting quietly and paying attention to one's breathing.

Try It: Sit quietly and comfortably. Close your eyes. Start by relaxing the muscles of your feet and work your way up your body, relaxing muscles as you go (a technique like Progressive Muscular Relaxation, described below, can be useful for this). Focus your attention on your breathing. Breathe in deeply and then let your breath out. Count your breaths, and say the number of the breath as you let it out (this gives you something to do with your mind, helping you to avoid distraction). Continue for ten to twenty minutes.

Progressive muscular relaxation is useful for relaxing tense muscles, and the effort can also help induce a greater state of calm. The idea is that by tensing your muscles first, you are able to relax them even more than you would otherwise.

Other tried and true techniques for reducing anxiety include

> **Try It:** Tense specific muscles as tightly as possible. Continue to strongly contract them for a moment or two, then relax. Finally, consciously relax the muscles even further, as far as you can.

quiet exercise, such as tai chi and yoga, journaling, allowing yourself to cry, talking to a trusted friend about your feelings and fears, enjoying a good book or a hot bath, or listening to soothing music.

Managing Anxiety - The Payoff

"Being free of anxiety doesn't mean you're not worrying about your loved one," Cammy says. "It means the worry isn't taking over your life. It's not keeping you from finding the good in all of your hard work."

Free from the draining effects of anxiety, you feel more relaxed and calm. You are more capable of handling the surprises and challenges that caregiving throws at you. Sleep isn't as difficult, and a less anxious you has a positive effect on the moods of those around you.

Without the punishing effects of depression and anxiety, you are coming closer to being truly Energized. But you may also fall prey to other negative emotions that are common among caregivers. The chapters ahead will help Educate you about denial, guilt and anger, Empowering you to face and defeat them and move ahead with renewed Energy.

The GIBBONS FAMILY Scrapbook

*N*o family starts out wanting to be the authority on loving and caring for someone with Alzheimer's disease. At least mine didn't. Even if we're not experts, we have sure learned some things along the crooked and sometimes treacherous road to the knowledge that we now wear as a badge of honor on our hearts and as frustration, born of a trial by fire, in our souls. Now that we have given you the best professional advice we can, I wanted to give you some thoughts from my family about what we learned and how we survived. —LEEZA GIBBONS

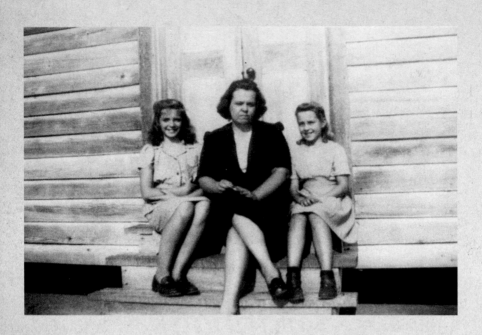

Granny and her girls! My Mom and Aunt Wayne. Must have been hard work parenting them judging from her expressions.

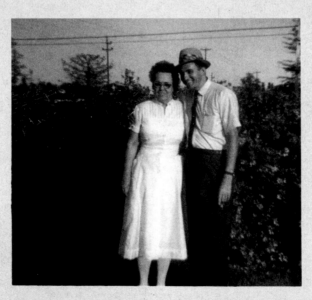

Daddy and Granny. Everyone loved Granny, Daddy too.
They teased each other all the time.

When you First Hear the News...

The first reaction is "this can't be true". There's a feeling of uncertainty, apprehension, anxiety, questions like where do I turn, what do I do, is there any help anywhere and how will this affect our lives, come pouring down on you all at one time and it's difficult to find a sense of normalcy. You just keep going, and know that somehow you'll get through. —*CARLOS, SR.*

Even if you suspect the worst, it still hurts like hell when you find out for sure. It's hard not to shriek "No!" and run out of the room or gasp and try desperately to change the conversation. It is a moment when you will feel as though you've been stripped of the ability to think logically. Wait. Listen. Then fall apart. If you know you are going to get a diagnosis, take someone with you to the appointment and don't make plans for anything afterwards. Chances are it will be hard to focus once that diagnosis has stripped all the oxygen out of the room. When we got Mom's diagnosis, we all went to lunch with her while it sank in. You will need time to let the news settle in. Mom was right when she said, "Don't hide it". Tell your friends, co-workers and family. You will need all of them during your journey. Keep notes of suggestions and advice; it will start coming in droves. Eliminate those people from your life who are uncomfortable, try to place blame or just drain you of energy (you will have enough to do without trying to manage or salvage these "vampire" relationships). —*LEEZA*

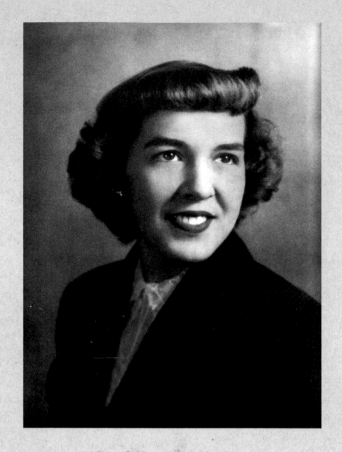

Jean Gibbons around age 20.
She did my hair like this once — it didn't look good on me either.

Breathe. A diagnosis like this will steal your breath away, leaving a lump in your throat that will threaten to choke you with the love and fear you will be feeling. Hold your family close to you. Physically hold them. You will bolster one another during the times to come, and this is just the beginning. Try your best to be brave in front of the one who has been diagnosed. Don't let your fear become his. Pray. Cry with your friends and family, and offer hope to your loved one, even when you may feel there is none. Do your research and ask all the questions you can think of before the answers slip away. Drop your expectations at the door. This is a process for you as much as it is for your loved one. —*CAMMY*

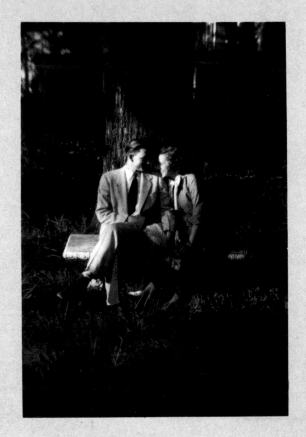

So in love...
Mom and Dad on the day they announced their engagement.

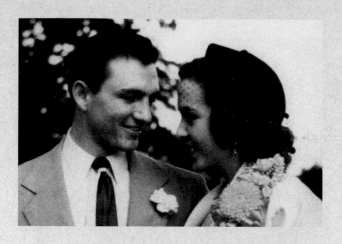

We've only just begun…
Mom and Dad on their wedding day.

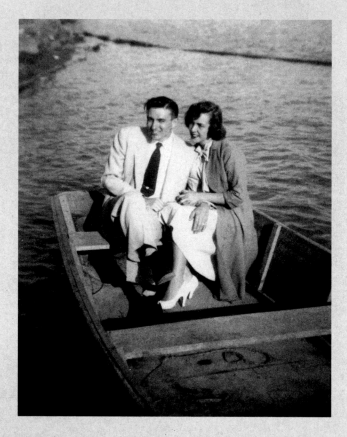

Still in their teens, Mom hangs on to her man, my Father.
High heels for her, a necktie for him—pretty fancy for a row boat.

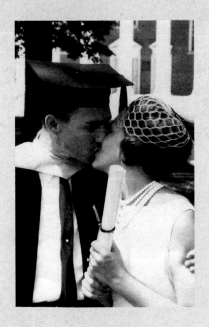

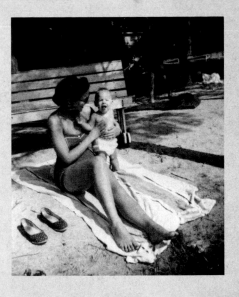

Dad gets his PhD.

*Bathing beauties. Mom and Carlos, Jr.
She was always happy with her arms
around a baby!*

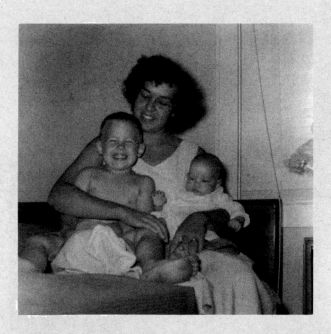

Arms full of joy! My brother Carlos and me safe in Mommy's embrace.

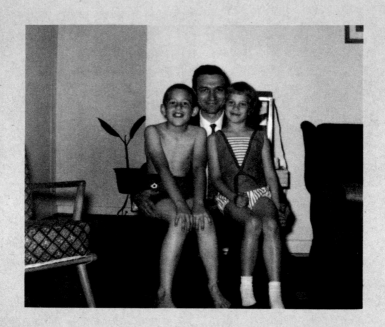

Daddy with Carlos and me. Notice we were each on one of his knees—he gave great "bouncy horsey" rides!

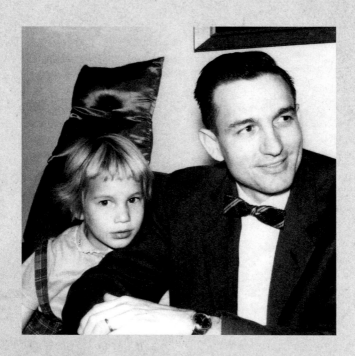

Daddy's girl. That's me with Dad at work. I loved going to the office.

You cannot be prepared for what will come next, so don't try to be. No one progresses at the same rate or with the same symptoms, so accept the situation, people and relationships in your life as they are. Treasure them, embrace them and value them. Be open, give yourself time to adapt to life as it evolves and let go of the desire to control it. Love, laugh and just be with those who matter to you as much as you can. —*ANNE MARIE*

Hang On To Hope...

Without hope there would be no other way to cope with something as devastating as Alzheimer's disease. If you have no hope, you can have no future. Even in the face of adversity, you have to cling to hope. One of the thoughts that has helped me through life is "Success is getting up one more time than you fall". When Alzheimer's comes into your life, you fall, but you have to get up. Hang on to hope even as you look into an uncertain future. —*CARLOS, SR.*

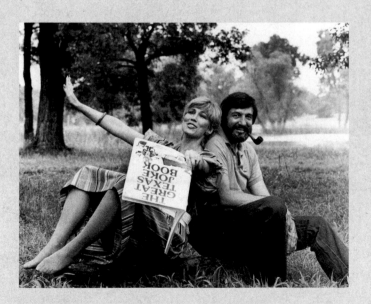

One of my favorite things to do with Daddy—telling jokes.
Shortly after this photo was taken he gave up his pipe.
The beard continued to make cameo appearances in his life.

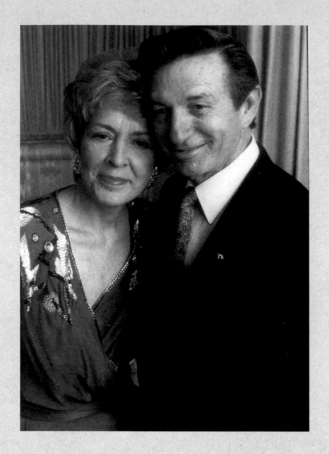

A Reflective Moment For Mom And Dad.

There will be plenty of doom and gloom. By now you have probably scoured the Internet to find every morsel of information that
may help you, and you might think that the cupboard is bare and the
prognosis is hopeless. Don't buy it. There are plenty of moments to
celebrate and the possibility of a miracle is always right around the
corner. That's how it happens, and it could happen for you. Some
may tell you this isn't realistic. But I never see the upside of negative,
defeatist thinking. I remember Mom becoming excited every time I
would read some encouraging news to her or give her a vitamin that
might help, or tell her about a new exercise class. The disease will
progress quickly or slowly, but it will progress. I don't say that to be
brutal, I say that to encourage you to consider that this is the time
to put on a new pair of glasses and try to see it differently. Rose is an
underrated color. —*LEEZA*

Believe in miracles and the promise that research provides. Do your best to look at "the big picture" and remind yourself that you don't know the answers to everything. Remind yourself that the answers may never come, and find a way to accept that. Celebrate every small moment, for it is within these small moments that you will find hope. When Mom could no longer speak, the days that she could curl her fingers around mine were miraculous. —*CAMMY*

Memories Matter Most Right Now...

The memories that mean most to me are the pleasant memories of dancing, taking trips, traveling, meeting friends, playing bridge and being a part of our community. Those things have been a great source of comfort to me. I can recall the days from the past 55 years of our marriage, but we have to remember that what we have is today and we can always choose to make a memory of right here , right now. I cherish the memories of spending time with Jean and feeding her even as she slipped away. Don't chase the tough times away from your roster of fond memories. You will be grateful for them even if you can't see it now. —*CARLOS, SR.*

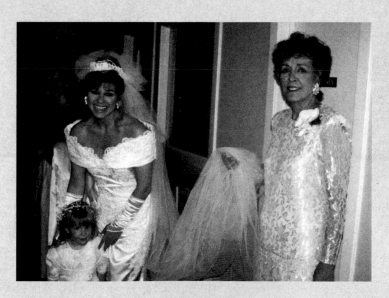

*Cammy's wedding day. Three of my favorite women—
my sister Cam, my Mom, and my daughter Lexi.*

I don't believe that memory exists solely in the brain. We are creatures ruled mostly by our hearts and I have always believed that a heart never forgets and is never forgotten. Hold onto your memories and pass them down, however you can. This new and uncomfortable chapter will still be a part of your story. Don't run from it, and don't believe that this is how the story ends. —*CAMMY*

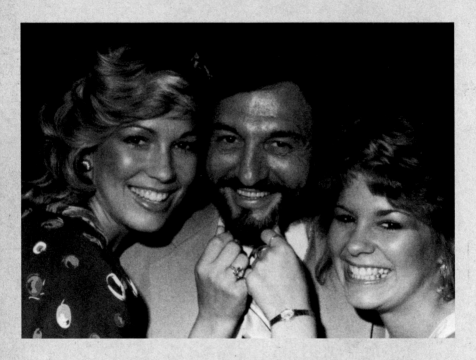

Cammy detests this picture but I love it! I'll argue with her about it later.

This is perhaps the most difficult part of your ordeal. One day your loved one seems present and connected and the next minute he or she is irrational and irritable. One day it may take 15 minutes to feed lunch and the next day it might be an hour. Everyone makes mistakes, but dwelling on them just makes it harder for both of you. Worrying about what will decline next, or wishing you could recapture something from the past will only prevent you from being in the present moment. Even as flawed and difficult as it may be, that is where life is. —*CARLOS, SR.*

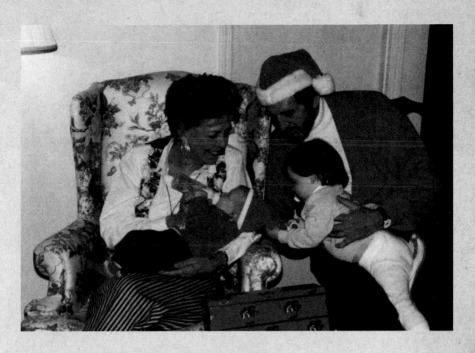

Mom never smiled brighter than when she was with her grandkids.
This was Lexi's first christmas and little Taylor was there to show her the way.
Dad always wore the Santa hat, a tradition I've continued.

If you haven't already said something you regret to the loved one with Alzheimer's disease, believe me, you will! It's frustrating, tiring and in many ways it's like developing a new relationship with someone you barely know. Forgive yourself. You are doing your best to keep up in a game where the rules are changing daily. Let go of expectations of yourself and your loved one. You can't be the patient, perfect caregiver all the time. Your loved one may become aggressive, event violent. There may be profanity. I remember Mom telling me, "When I kick and scream and call you names, know that is the disease talking, not me." I can't think of any better advice. Look past the behavior to the person underneath, who can no longer find a way to come out. There will come a time when even the difficult behavior you face today may seem like a gift. Focus on what you can do right now-today. Sing, hold hands, brush hair. Record the voice of the one who is disappearing. You'll be surprised how comforting it is to have when or if your loved one goes silent before the end. —*LEEZA*

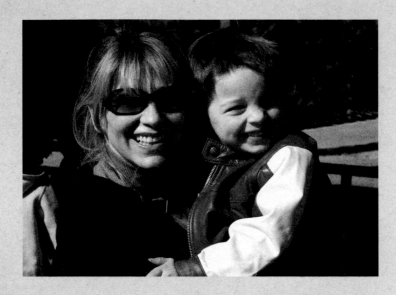

Cammy and her favorite person in the whole world, her son Blake.
The older he gets, the more he looks like her, inlcuding the mischevious grin.

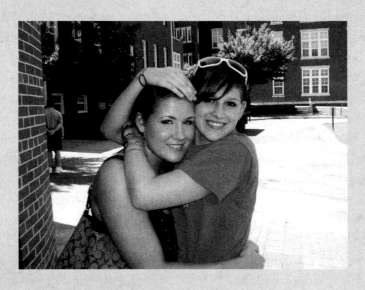

My beautiful nieces Kelly and Taylor.

This is the great unknown, which is scary for everyone. But imagine how scary it must be for the one experiencing this ravaging disease. We can't possibly understand. So we must be the support and comfort for our loved one day by day, minute by minute. Embrace and accept what is now. There were times when I knew that Jean had no idea what was going on in the world or even in her room, but when I walked in with kindness, comfort and no expectations, I felt that there was some place deep inside of her that instinctively felt my love for her. Be gentle, forgiving and understanding. —*ANNE MARIE*

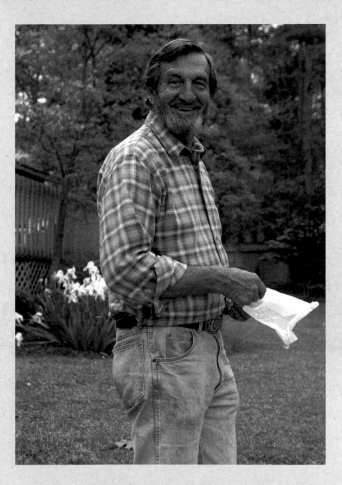

One of my favorite pictures of Daddy—
casual and relaxed with that warm smile of his.

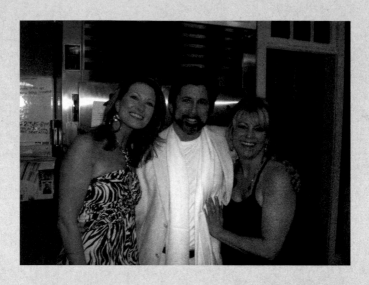

Three of my favorite people Anne Marie, known as Contessa, Dr. J. (my inspiration and our co-author) and the Empress, my sis, Cam (by the way, I am The Queen).

My brother Carlos, my sister-in-law Anne Marie and my neice Kelly.

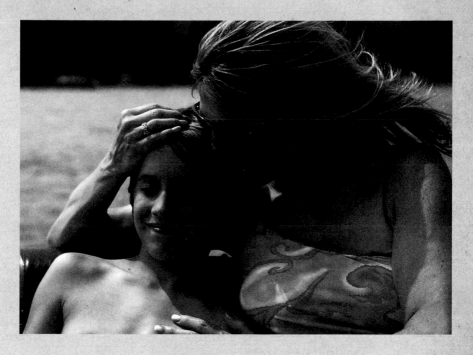

I melt every time I see this picture. Troy and I were on Lake Murray
enjoying a sunny summer day on the back of the pontoon boat as
Daddy proudly escorted us around his domain.

God bless my sister for insisting on preparing for the time when
Mom could no longer make decisions for herself. There may be
a part of you that doesn't want to take care of the arrangements;
it feels too much like letting go. I had been charged with writing Mom's obituary for years before she died; I only completed it
three days before it actually happened. The truth is, no one wants
to say goodbye. Even knowing that death would offer her a free-
dom and escape, I did not want to let go. Mom gave us a gift beyond measure in detailing her wishes. Do that now, as much as it
hurts. There is comfort in knowing you have honored your loved
one as best you can. Never stop saying "I love you." No one knows
what a person in the final stages of Alzheimer's disease can hear or
comprehend. Believe that you are communicating by heart, and
do the best you can. —*CAMMY*

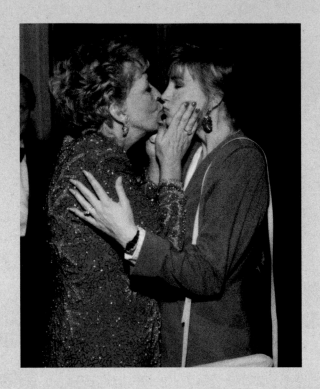

A kiss for luck from my mom. I have this same picture with my daughter—minus the long fingernails.

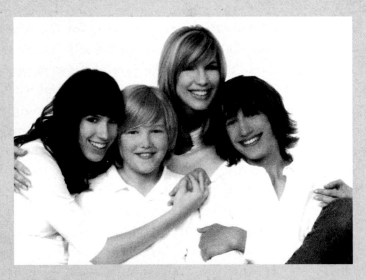

Lexi, Nathan and Troy, the heart and soul of all that I do. Love trancends time and space. We will be together forever.

Let's face it: none of us wants to confront the death of someone we love. It's easy to let time go by without ever discussing plans, wishes and desires. But if you can get your family together, it will turn out to be a huge blessing and probably save sanity and expense.

My "Steel Magnolia" mom was rare in giving us strict instructions for her care, and we were so grateful that she did. Mom said, "When I can no longer call you by name, I don't want to live with any of you kids and you'll have to help Daddy let me go." She even told us the kind of place she wanted to go when she couldn't be at home! None of this surprised me; Mom told me years before her diagnosis that she wanted to be buried in her pajamas (a request we granted!). The truth is, we never fought about what was best for Mom. We had her exact wishes as our guide. Consider having your loved one do a "Wish List" about how she wants to be cared for. This way, she will not feel left out when the time comes to make these decisions and the family can all move in the same direction. Does she want to be read to? Does she want someone to hold her hand? Of course, there will be more pragmatic decisions to be made, like preparing a durable power of attorney and a living will. If you can handle this during the early stage of the disease that is best, since your loved one may lose cognitive ability later on making the process much more difficult. —*LEEZA*

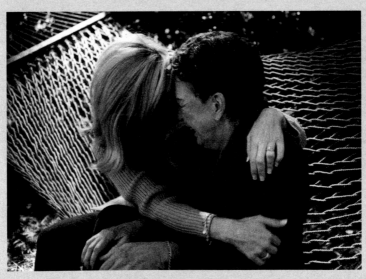

Mom has wrapped her arms around me so many times. How lucky for me that I had the chance to embrace her on this day when she still remembered who I was.

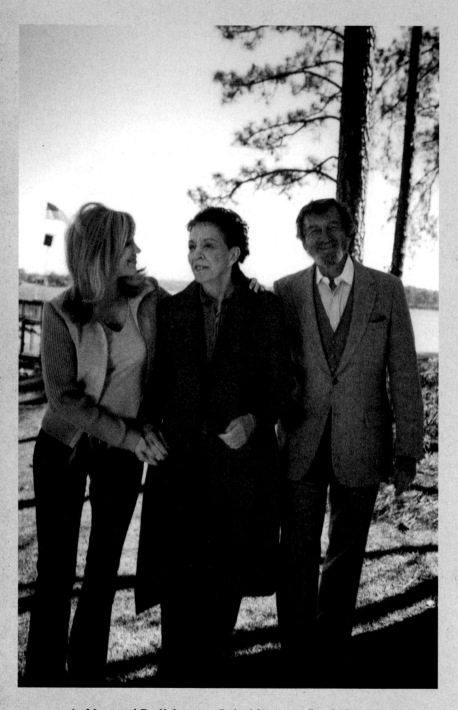

At Mom and Dad's house at Lake Murray in South Carolina.
Alzheimer's had given mom a slightly dazed look, but she held
her head high, boldly claiming her disease.

CHAPTER 8

Overcoming Denial and Guilt

Leeza: No one wants to accept the loss of someone they love. When my mom began to show signs of Alzheimer's disease, our family was in denial. We were content to say to ourselves, "Mom's losing it." Our family, like most families facing this disease, had blinders on.

To experience life is to experience constant change. As Leeza'a family found, change can be frightening and painful, and some of the hardest changes we'll ever deal with come when a loved one is diagnosed with a memory loss disorder. It means he cannot function as he once did, cannot be depended on to be the same person we have always known, and may not even remember us for very much longer. To the caregiver, facing these changes means giving up familiar routines, adapting to increasing limitations and most of all letting go of someone we love, little by little. It's a difficult process that is frequently made harder by two internal obstacles: *denial* and *guilt*.

Denial

Lexi : I have a hard time thinking about denial because I never know if I'm in it or not. I believe sometimes I react to many aspects of life in general with denial. I always believed that if I didn't think about whatever the subject might be, it wouldn't be real, so I always thought about J.G.'s Alzheimer's as something that would go away. I never stepped back to think about any of it.

I'm the oldest of the kids in a family that was attacked head-on by this awful disease. So I took the position of "steady and calm." I thought I had to. I had two younger brothers. So I acted as therapist, sister, daughter, father, and whatever else was needed from me, all willingly of course. My first reaction to anything my family needs is to be there, so I never really thought about if I was dealing with it myself until the day J.G. passed away. That day, all of these crazy thoughts and feelings swept into me and again, my first reaction was complete denial. I focused on the songs I had to sing at the funeral, I made sure I was perfect for her so that wherever she was, J.G. would be proud of me. But I still, to this day, have not really dealt with the diagnosis, the escalation of the disease, or J.G.'s death and funeral. And it was only when I started to write this that I even realized that.

As caregivers, our lives sometimes seem to be running us rather than the other way around. We want to feel in control again. One Leeza's Place client described feeling "as though I'm stuck in a car without a steering wheel." Many of us respond (perhaps unconsciously) to this lack of control by resisting reality, as if by resisting what we do not like we can take charge of our lives again. At first, we might deny that the disease even exists: we might avoid getting a diagnosis; we might keep to rigid routines and refuse to make way for the unplanned and unwanted course of the disease, all in an effort to "prevent" it from really happening. But in the end, resisting only increases our suffering and keeps us from real happiness and inner peace.

Denial, a natural response to the fear of change, is one of the primary ways we resist the all-important acceptance of reality and complicate our already complicated lives. Denial is often turned to in times of great stress. When our lives take a sudden turn for the worse, when tragedy comes into our homes and threatens our way of life, when we are faced with any serious loss, we might choose denial as a way of coping. Just like the "blinders" Leeza referred to, denial screens out information we aren't prepared to accept.

Elisabeth Kübler-Ross, the eminent psychiatrist and author of *On Death and Dying,* lists denial as one of the five stages of grief a person passes thorough in accepting the death of a loved one, as when parents, on being informed of the accidental death of a child, will say, "No! You must have the wrong address, it can't be our baby." This kind of denial is usually short-term, eventually discarded when the person has had time to deal with the new reality. In this form, it is a natural and important coping mechanism in tragic situations.

Short-term denial can occur on a small scale, blurring over an unsettling event or change so that we don't *quite* see it in its frightening entirety (and so have no need to accept it as it is), such as our loved one's failure to remember us. Or it can occur on a large scale, such as when we deny the existence of the disease entirely. We may choose to believe that the disease was misdiagnosed, is not so serious, or that our loved one seems to be improving. When we use denial as a way of coping temporarily, it can be a lifesaver and give us time to gain enough strength to face reality.

But when denial prevents us from facing reality for an extended period of time or hinders us from taking action when needed, it is considered unhealthy and dangerous. When Mom insists that her vegetarian son "loves steak," it might frustrate him and create conflict, but it's not especially harmful. When denial takes root in more serious situations, it may generate enormous pain and delay important responses. Imagine that same mom finds drugs in her son's clothes, but insists that "they can't be his" and lets the matter go by quietly. Her denial of the painful reality—that her son uses drugs—keeps her from taking action that might help her son, and also erodes the intimacy between them. How can we be close with someone if we are in denial about what he is doing or who he is?

When a memory disorder such as Alzheimer's disease is diagnosed, caregivers often retreat into denial, along with their loved ones. Sometimes denial begins as early as when the first symptoms become apparent. Many people have obvious symptoms of Alzheimer's disease, for example, but its victims and their caregivers put off getting a diagnosis, instead insisting that the symptoms are a sign of normal aging or that the changes in behavior are due to stress at work or at home. In either case, denial prevents an early diagnosis and precious time is lost for planning or seeking out the best therapies.

In other instances, caregivers might live in denial of their true feelings. You may want to think of yourself as a nice, loving husband, when in reality you are angry or hurt by the gradual loss of your loved one, but you are unwilling to accept such negative feelings about yourself and so deny their existence entirely. Denial is different from *consciously lying* about our feelings. It goes deeper. With denial, we're lying to ourselves by denying reality. Denial goes beyond blinders and makes us deaf as well: we rarely hear what others are trying to tell us. If confronted about our denial, we might respond with shock and indignation. We can actually believe that we are "fine", when everyone and everything around us suggests otherwise.

WAKING UP FROM DENIAL

Denial can be overcome in three steps – what we call *recognition*, *education*, and *resolution*. First, we must *recognize* that denial exists and we must want to break free from it. This isn't as simple as it sounds. We may find that we prefer denial to facing reality. If we have emotions that we don't wish to have, giving up denial means we have to experience those unwanted emotions. But once we *educate* ourselves and accept that denial is not an effective way to deal with reality, that it actually increases our pain and misery, we learn that there are better ways to cope. We then realize that *resolving* denial is an important step towards living a full and satisfying life.

We can begin overcoming denial by learning what denial looks like in our lives. See if you recognize in yourself any of these signs of denial:

- You feel as though you are in a daze, going through the motions of dealing with life, are easily distracted, and do not fully perceive things around you.
- You are concocting fantasies to explain what has happened. You are misinterpreting what others are saying or doing.
- You are less efficient, and small tasks appear very complicated. You are obsessing about minor details and avoiding larger responsibilities.
- Your emotions are blocked or numbed. You feel mechanical or you may explode easily, taking you and others by surprise.
- You suffer from a variety of unexplained aches and pains.
- You are avoiding situations or feelings that remind you of an unpleasant reality. For example, you avoid loving feelings towards your sick spouse, because you will be reminded of your grief.

If you recognize that denial is playing a part in your life, you can begin to address it more directly and sort out what is being denied. Overcoming denial requires a constant commitment to face what you are afraid of. You need to reverse the unconscious decision that awareness of certain feelings, needs, or thoughts is more threatening to your sense of self than is the act of denial. While you are in the process of struggling through denial, you can actively work to increase your self-esteem and thereby encourage your ability to handle reality. Ways in which you we can help yourself increase self-esteem include:

- Self-Acceptance. Is just that, despite our perceived weakness es and failings. It is avoiding perfectionism and instead ac cepting that you are doing the best you can.
- Rethinking Values. A memory loss disorder changes every thing. Rethinking values means adjusting what you have believed to your new reality.
- Tuning out Negative Self-Talk. When you expect bad news, you hear bad news. When you are told that all is lost, all will seem to be lost. Be aware of negativity in the way you approach your daily life, and work on seeing as much of the positive as you can in any situation.

Leeza's Place has developed a program called Picture Yourself, a video tool that enables a caregiver to serve as her own "life coach" in developing a better sense of self esteem. During the program (which can be done at home), the caregiver gathers motivational materials such as saying and pictures and symbols of her own personal happiness, such as her favorite flowers and music. The caregiver then incorporates these items with a written narrative extolling her own positive qualities, such as her spirituality, loyalty, and forgiving nature. The caregiver then speaks directly into the camera, describing her own positive personal qualities that others may or may not be aware of. Not only does the exercise allow the caregiver to immediately remind herself of her own value, she has a permanent video that she can revisit each time in her caregiving life that she needs a boost to her self esteem.

Banishing Denial - The Payoff

"With our 'blinders' off," Leeza says, "We were free to respond to our situation in an effective and timely way. We were more aware of our own emotions, and more aware of Mom's feelings – everyone's feelings, really. Honest and effective communication among us and our doctors flowed more easily, leaving us feeling more connected and capable of facing our caregiving roles."

Guilt

Cammy: I think we avoided a lot of the guilt many families feel when a loved one gets seriously ill and the family doesn't know if they are doing all they can to help and, more importantly, if they are doing as their loved one would have wanted, particularly when a decision has to be made about placement in a care facility. We were lucky, in a sense, because Mom knew what was wrong with her and she also knew she was going to get worse, and had given thought to what she wanted for herself. Just after her diagnosis, Mom gathered everyone around her and said, "When I kick and scream and call you names, know that it is the disease talking. It is not me. And when I no longer know that you are my daughters, my son and my husband, that is the time that I no longer want to live with you. Leeza, I know you're gonna try to fix it, but I don't want to live with you, or your sister or your brother and you're all going to have to help Daddy let me go."

As a family we reflected on that often. It saved us from the internal fighting that often occurs where one sibling thinks they know best, or the siblings are trying to move the other parent in a particular direction. We had our marching orders and as difficult as they were, we carried them out.

But, I don't think you can ever avoid all the guilt. I remember after Mom was admitted to the nursing home, they wouldn't let Dad see her for the first five days so that they could work on getting her to adjust to her new surroundings. That was tough on Dad. Then when they did allow us in, at first they only let us observe her without her knowing we were there. It was heartbreaking, to see how much work they had to put in to try to keep her calm. I'm sure Mom was just frightened out of her wits, not knowing where she was and not having any familiar faces around her. There were times during those first days when we just wanted to take her away from there, but we remembered what Mom had told us she wanted and in the end, I think we did the right thing.

I know Leeza had her own tough time dealing with the fact that she lived and worked so far away from the family. I think it was scary for her. She once told me that it was much easier to write a check or make a phone call than to be the hands-on person who was witnessing this daily decline. It ended up making her feel powerless, frustrated and guilty that she couldn't do everything that needed to be done for Mom and the family when she was 3,000 miles away.

You may have experienced the feelings that Cammy describes: deep feelings born of love, pain and helplessness. On some level, you may even feel responsible for the disease afflicting your loved one. You may feel that perhaps you didn't catch it early enough, or that you didn't love your parent or spouse as much as you should have when they were healthy. You may berate yourself for your perceived failures rather than focusing on the good you achieve. If this is the case, you are suffering from one of the most common—and one of the most debilitating—emotional difficulties faced by caregivers: *guilt*.

Guilt is a paralyzing emotion arising from one's inability to accept oneself or a situation. It can lead to frustration, depression and other emotional problems. Guilt is usually a negative focus upon oneself: "I am an evil person. I can't bear myself. I am unworthy." At its core, guilt is linked to low self-esteem. We believe we are wrong or bad in some way, that we aren't doing enough, we aren't feeling the way we should, or we simply aren't good.

The qualities listed above may lead to frequent guilt, and frequent guilt may lead to these qualities; it can become a never-ending cycle. A Leeza's Place client, Patty, experienced firsthand how guilt arising from caregiving could come to dominate her life. Patty's father moved in with her and her family shortly after he was diagnosed with Parkinson' disease. Her husband Alan, a family doctor, worked long and erratic hours and Patty was already taking care of three children.

The strain of caregiving was taking its toll on the entire family, but Patty couldn't bring herself to put her father in the hands of a stranger after all the years he had spent as a single parent caring for her and her sister. Time went by and Patty was constantly fatigued, coming down with every cold that passed her way and snapping at the kids more and more often. As her father's need for assistance grew, she felt she could never do enough for him or the family. She became frustrated when her efforts to try to "fix" things for her father created conflicts in her own life, and unfortunately the fixes never seemed to last. Ultimately, she felt she was losing control of her life.

Her conflicting priorities led to feelings of helplessness and guilt. This self-imposed guilt then became her constant companion. She grew more exhausted than ever and increasingly withdrawn, and it was a vicious cycle: her low self-esteem (I can't do what I am "supposed" to do, e.g. take care of Dad and three kids on my own) led to feeling guilty, which led to increased negativity about herself, which again led to more guilt.

Feelings of guilt can be self-inflicted or can be pushed upon us by other people. In our culture, guilt is often designed to influence our behavior: "If you loved me you would do what I want." "Fine, do what you want and forget about your poor mother." Guilt can be passed on from generation to generation, sometimes through religion, often through families. When guilt is legitimate, it can spur us to do better. But this is short-term guilt, easily resolved by action.

IF YOU FEEL GUILTY FREQUENTLY, YOU MAY FIND THAT YOU ALSO HAVE ONE OR MORE OF THE FOLLOWING EMOTIONAL CHARACTERISTICS:

- Low self-esteem.
- Perfectionist tendencies.
- An inability to let go of anger (at yourself or others).
- An inability to forgive others who have wronged you.
- A tendency to be depressed.
- Frequent anxiety.
- A need to be in control.

Unhealthy guilt that lingers without resolution only causes anxiety and hinders one's ability to live one's life in peace, to make sound decisions and deliver quality care. We must be able to distinguish between legitimate guilt that motivates us to do better and harmful guilt that might be undeserved and that leaves us dispirited and ultimately incapable of doing all we can for our loved ones.

Kelly (age 17): I am J.G.'s third grandchild, after Taylor and Lexi. I'm kind of a free spirit, and my Mom tells me that is how J.G. used to be, so I kind of identify with her. I remember feeling guilty about not going to see J.G. when she was in the nursing home. I didn't want to see her because I didn't want to watch this happen to her and because I didn't want to remember her like that. We would go there every holiday. I didn't want to go inside. Mom didn't make me because she said that J.G. had a hard time going to see her own mother when she was in the nursing home, so she didn't want to force me to do something J.G. hadn't wanted to do herself. I remember everyone coming out of the nursing home and they'd all be so upset, and I'd hear the reports that she was getting worse. Because she and I have so much in common and she's one of my favorite people in the world, I didn't want to lose that memory of her. I wanted to remember her the way she was.

Caregivers are prone to guilt for many reasons. Few people fully understand the complexities of the health problems suffered by our loved ones, or the insurance coverage, senior housing, drug plan, Medicare, legal and other senior-related issues that need to be faced, and we sometimes make mistakes or simply feel incompetent—both of which lead to guilt. If we are caring for a parent, we are not prepared for the change in roles and new responsibilities the job brings.

Uninformed friends and family may offer help, but often their attempts serve to highlight our lack of confidence and shortcomings, which makes us feel guilty. Others might want to impose guilt upon us. Real or perceived failures in our caregiving obligations can lead to criticism, though that criticism is often from family members who do far less than we do, but who want to pass their guilt on.

CONQUERING GUILT

Leaving guilt behind ultimately means accepting who you are and where you are in life. If you don't, you are simply not able to take care of your loved ones or yourself effectively. You must feel confident that you've done your best. You need to *practice* accepting who you are and valuing yourself enough to overcome the guilt of perceived inadequacy. Perfectionism and the need to be in control may be major roadblocks to overcoming guilt, so you may need to learn to let go of these tendencies first.

But there's no easy remedy for guilt, no quick fix. Freeing yourself from guilt is an ongoing process, one that you must attend to every day so that you can successfully reclaim your life and your energy. Ways in which you can facilitate this process include:

- Get the help of a therapist. The act of discussing your feelings out loud can be an important step towards self-forgiveness.
- Determine if the guilt is warranted. Ask yourself if everything has been done that is practical and necessary within reasonable limits. Often the caregiver struggles to meet the ever-increasing needs of their loved one at great personal sacrifice, and berates herself for not doing more.
- Write down the things that make you feel guilty. Examine

the underlying reasons for your guilt and determine if there are changes that can be made.

- Break down large problems into smaller issues. This can make them seem more manageable. Resolving a few problems can give you a sense of accomplishment and build your confidence to handle those never-ending new surprises as they arise.
- Concentrate on what can be done now. It is never helpful to punish yourself about the past. Resist the temptation to allow old conflicts to create guilt today.

Beyond Guilt - The Payoff

You won't overcome guilt in a day. If you have a tendency towards guilt, you'll need to use these tools on a regular basis to accept and learn from your mistakes. But imagine your life without guilt. Imagine how you'd feel about yourself if you didn't regret your mistakes. Practice letting go. Practice forgiveness. If you allow yourself to recognize when you feel guilty, the caregiving process can be less draining and more fulfilling. When you are no longer burdened by guilt, your energy returns and you can meet the challenges with renewed vitality and strength.

CHAPTER 9

Managing Anger

*C*ammy: *Tonight I am initialing Mom's socks with a brand new Sharpie – it has to be a Sharpie, everything else washes out – and I am upset because her name has run inside the tenth pair of socks I've done. I wonder why I get so angry about it, why I want her name to be perfect; after all, no one will see these socks except for us and maybe a few others and they seem to disappear at an alarming rate anyhow. I've noticed that the more "wearable" clothes that I buy for her have a way of disappearing fast too. I try not to think about that as I make a point to say thank you to those who care for her. They make next to nothing and they work so hard doing all of the things that I, her daughter, should be doing for her, but I just can't. I hate that about myself. I am weak and Mom deserves more from me, but I just can't.*

I still need her to be my Mom. So I can't ever change her diapers. God forgive me, but I just can't. So if the gals who do that for me and for her, if they call her by name and are kind to her, if they can take her cursing and hitting on the way to the shower, if those gals want to cop a few Jaclyn Smith elastic pants and tops from Kmart, well, I'm not ever going complain.

I can't even seem to initial her socks without feeling like I've somehow let her down, because I can't find a way to save

*her from living out what she feared all of her life. I purpose-
fully don't go to see her so much anymore. It's been six years
now and it never did get any easier, going to see her in a place
to which I promised I would never send her. My only comfort
is in knowing that she knew where she was headed, and she
dreaded it more for me than even I dread it now. Mom had already walked in my shoes, watching her mother slip away into
an unknowable, vacant, embarrassing stranger. She wanted
me to promise that I would never go to see her like that if she
had to go to a home. I never could make that promise. Neither
could my brother and sister. How could we?*

*I think about what good friends we were and how I would
have liked to have known her when her footsteps were im-
printing the ground that I'm trying to balance on now. With
every step I take, I realize how brave she had to be to take
another step. Tomorrow we'll talk about her new haircut and
how great she looks as I put away her new socks and slip-
pers, trying not to wince at the pair in which her initials got
smeared into a blur, and I will cry as I leave and go on with
my day. Just like always. Just like she did. I think I may get
a label machine for the socks. Maybe a Bedazzler, too. She'd
like that.*

Anger is normal, and healthy when experienced appropriately.
Faced with the many frustrations of caregiving, it's expected that
we will get angry. It could happen for many reasons: sometimes our
best efforts don't seem to be enough; our loved one doesn't appreciate us or even recognize us. We might feel like we are the only one
who is trying to help, or we are just angry that the disease is part
our life and is stealing our loved one. Sometimes, however, anger
becomes a problem. It can become a chronic condition affecting us

both physically and emotionally, and affecting the lives of our loved one and everyone else around us. If we understand when anger is reasonable and when anger is unhealthy, we can better manage anger during the difficulties that come with caregiving.

Some anger can be an important motivator for change, such as anger at injustice or cruelty. This kind of anger fuels efforts to make the world a better place. Anger can also give us strength to make difficult personal changes. Many therapists believe that anger is one of the most powerful motivating factors in successful therapy, providing the courage a person needs for change.

Anger arises in response to both internal and external problems. It can result from a belief that we've been harmed, or from feelings of powerlessness. When we feel threatened, we often respond in anger to keep the world at a distance and protect ourselves. Anger also works as a defense against unwanted emotions. It may be used to mask feelings of inadequacy or vulnerability, to feel stronger and cover up our fear. Anger may be used to deflect hurt feelings or guilt: we might get angry to divert attention away from these other, more painful feelings.

As common as the experience of anger is, most of us have not been taught how to deal with anger in a positive way. The failure to acknowledge and experience our anger can disrupt relationships, affect thinking and behavior patterns and affect us physically, causing high blood pressure, heart problems, headaches, and digestive disorders. Some experts believe that suppressed anger is an underlying cause of both anxiety and depression. When anger becomes a problem, we get upset easily or feel irritable all the time. Anger can be contagious: the entire family can be affected by the tension anger creates. In such an environment, communication becomes strained, and emotional and physical abuses are more likely to occur.

Instead of just feeling the anger and letting it go, we sometimes feel guilty about it and suppress it as best we can. We say things to ourselves that only make the problem worse, like, "I can't be angry with him when he's sick," or, "If I was a better daughter I wouldn't feel this angry." We think getting angry means that there must be something wrong with us, and our self-esteem drops down another notch. The cycle continues without ever allowing anger to fully surface. But our true kindness, our "loving heart," as the author and Buddhist nun Pema Chodron put it, "is not even a possibility unless we attend to our own demons."

And what a demon anger can be! When you repress any emotion, you are not being honest. Repression threatens connections between people and creates isolation. Being able to recognize unhealthy anger means you can channel its destructive power and integrate it into your life in a positive way. You can choose to end the spiral of guilt and low self esteem that repressed anger causes. Embracing even your most difficult feelings can give you the peace of mind that comes from being true to yourself.

Working Through the Anger

How can we make peace with this difficult emotion? The antidote to our anger problem is two-fold: first, we need to give ourselves permission to experience it as immediately and completely as possible. Our inability to experience anger immediately causes it to gain power and take a stronger hold, turning it into resentment or depression. If we just *allow it*, anger will not poison our lives and we will not waste valuable energy fighting it. Second, we need to address our own sense of low self worth. The lower our self-esteem, the greater our tendency towards guilt, which increases our anger. Consider the following strategies for managing your anger:

Practice acceptance. It's okay to feel angry. It's okay to feel angry with our loved ones when they are sick. It's okay to be angry, even when it doesn't "make sense." It is also okay to be unable to "let go" of all our anger, as long as we are committed to paying attention to it and not avoiding it.

Educate yourself. If you aren't aware of how your loved one's disease manifests itself, you may become resentful of its symptoms or try to correct behaviors over which your loved one has no control. Accept that you have to join the person in his world because he can't join you in yours.

Communicate anger effectively. Asserting your feelings clearly can help you to feel better about yourself and increase your self-control in everyday situations.

Recognize anger when it arises. One way to do this it to pay attention to its physical manifestation. Anger, like all emotions, is a physical experience as well as an emotional one. Our heart rate increases, we feel hotter, our throat gets tighter, our head feels like it's going to burst. We often don't even have to *do* anything with our anger in order to reduce it; sometimes just realizing it is there can help.

Let go of expectations. Expectations create anxiety and judgment. We worry about what is going to happen tomorrow or berate ourselves over what occurred yesterday. Remember - now is the most vital, important moment.

Yield to the universe. Give in to the reality that we lack power over everything. Explore different spiritualities, and systems that encourage self-growth. In the end, they are about letting go. If we struggle to control the world, we are setting ourselves up to be angry (see Chapter 11).

PRACTICE ASSERTIVENESS, NOT ANGER

- Be as specific and clear as possible about what you want, think, and feel. It can be helpful to explain exactly what you mean and exactly what you don't mean, such as "I don't want to put Mom in a home, but I'd like to have a little more support from the rest of the family."
- Be direct. Deliver your message to the person for whom it is intended. If you want to tell Mark something, tell Mark.
- Own your message. Acknowledge that your message comes from your frame of reference. You can acknowledge ownership with personalized ("I") statements such as "I don't agree with you" (as compared to "You're wrong") or "I'd like you to mow the lawn" (as compared to "You really should mow the lawn"). Suggesting that someone is wrong or bad and should change for his or her own benefit will only foster resentment and resistance rather than understanding and cooperation.
- Ask for feedback. "Am I being clear? How do you see this situation? What do you want to do?" Asking for feedback can encourage others to correct any misperceptions you may have as well as help others realize that you are expressing an opinion, feeling, or desire rather than a demand. Encourage others to be clear, direct, and specific in their feedback to you.

Managing Anger - the Payoff

"I'm so glad I've worked through the anger," Cammy says. "Sure, when I think about the long process of losing Mom there are plenty of things to be upset about, but not letting the negativity consume me lets me see the world as a better place. And it becomes much easier to deal with my feelings about Mom, too."

Caregiving can be the impetus for transforming yourself and your world in a positive way. We all need to take care of our emotional selves, just as we need to take care of our physical selves. Rather than continue to wear anger as a mask or repress it in fear, come to terms with it. Once you face your anger, you can release it and replace it with confidence and renewed energy.

Carlos, Sr.'s O2 for Caregivers

DEAL WITH YOUR ANGER

One thing Jean taught me was not to go to bed angry. But I guess anger is a natural part of caregiving. Here are some things that helped me deal with mine:

- Have no expectations because they lead to anger, disappointment and resentment.
- Don't take it personally. Don't get defensive. It may sound like it's about you, but it isn't. Recognize that the anger coming at you is based in grief or fear.
- Find constructive ways to channel your anger.

PART IV:

CARING FOR THE CAREGIVER'S SPIRIT

Life demands only the strength you possess. One feat is possible—not to have run away.

—Dag Hammarskjold

CHAPTER 10

Nourishing Your Family's Spirit—And Your Own

Troy: Walking into the room at the Alzheimer's hospital and seeing my grandma lying there with a dazed look on her face, as though she was focused on nothing was the most heartbreaking thing I can remember. When I first saw her there, I didn't quite understand it. She was there, I saw her, I knew she was in the room, but I didn't completely get why she didn't acknowledge the people coming into the room, or anything at all. She just looked at the same spot nearly the whole time we were in the room. She said nothing, moved every so often but not much, and just stared into the distance. I wanted to talk to her, ask her how she was doing, how things were, all of that stuff. But I couldn't. I look over at my mom and she was kneeling next to J.G., crying, talking to her. I wanted some way to fix it, some way that I could help, but I couldn't do anything. We talked with Grandma for a bit, but she still didn't speak. My mom was talking about back home and how things were and how we were all doing. She then mentioned Nathan and me, who were both in the room at the time. Suddenly, a sort of awareness came into J.G.'s eyes and facial expression. She said, "My sweet boys."

I sort of just stared in amazement. My mom looked at me,

then Nathan, back at me, then at her mom. Mom began to cry and said, "Yes mom, your sweet boys." I realized after that, that nothing could take J.G. away from us. I began to cry.

Caregiving doesn't just put a strain on the body and mind—it can drain your spirit as well. But at Leeza's Place, we've seen that the spirit can actually be strengthened by the work of caregiving. This is a reward that can be shared by your entire family, and as many of us know, a happy family can be a source of great strength during even the worst trials.

By involving other members of your family in the Three E's, you can reduce your burden and increase the joy that can be derived from caregiving, creating a "cycle of strength" that benefits everyone: you are energized by them, and they by you. And, of course, that energy translates into better care for your loved one and for yourself.

First, remember "E" Number 1: Education. Successfully caring for a person with a degenerative memory disorder requires that the whole family be involved, which means educating everyone about the disease and about what to expect in the future. Particular care must be taken to educate the youngest members of the family. Having a grandparent or other close relative develop a memory loss disorder can be particularly distressing for young children. But often, children aren't kept informed about the condition of a loved one and are left without the emotional resources to deal with the sudden change in their family. Children need to know why their loved one is changing, why her thinking and behavior may seem a bit strange. Be sure that children understand it is the disease causing the behaviors, and not the person.

Taylor: I think that feeling like you're being kept in the dark is the hardest part for grandchildren, especially for the younger ones. Particularly in the later stages it makes it hard if they don't know what's going on, and they don't know what they have to change about how they approach their grandparent. I remember thinking,"Why doesn't J.G. understand what I'm telling her about school?" Luckily, my mom was good about telling me what was happening. I'm sure that not everyone gets filled in on the details and it really does negatively impact their ability to interact with their loved one.

Encouraging open communication about feelings is essential. Open communication can be difficult for any family, but especially for one dealing with a memory disorder. Sometimes families avoid speaking about the disease, perhaps because there is still a great deal of stigma and fear attached to Alzheimer's disease and other memory disorders.

The spouse of one suffering from the disorder might wish to hide the disease from other family members to protect their spouse's (or their own) privacy and dignity. An adult child might keep the truth of the disease from his or her own children in an effort to "spare" them the pain. But secrets generate emotional distance and confusion, and the caregiver is more likely to become overwhelmed by trying to shoulder the burden alone. Sometimes family issues become so complicated that it might be necessary to seek the guidance of a family counselor. (In fact, as awareness of the special world of caregiving grows, a new counseling niche is emerging: the "caregiving coach").

As with the individual caregiver, an educated family is an empowered family. When your family has a better sense of what is happening around them during this difficult time, they know better how to respond. They can take a more active role in reducing your stress. In fact, an increasing number of caregiving parents report

**WHAT YOUR CHILD MAY BE FEELING
WHEN A FAMILY MEMBER IS SUFFERING
FROM ALZHEIMER'S DISEASE:**

- Grief, due to witnessing the losses the family member experiences.
- Shame, about your loved one's condition. She may avoid inviting friends home.
- Anxiety, if she detects stress in the parents' relationship.
- Loneliness, due to a parent focusing his or her attention on the ill family member.
- Awkwardness, due to a reversal of roles within the family.
- Frustration, due to changes in lifestyle.
- Fear, about their own future and their chances of getting Alzheimer's disease.

that their children are helping with many of the tasks associated with giving care to a loved one, from helping with cooking and cleaning to assisting with transportation and doctor's appointments. These caregivers also report that, as a result of their family's participation, the quality of the care they are giving has increased, along with their own feelings of personal satisfaction. We've all heard the expression, "there's strength in numbers," and nowhere is it so true as in caregiving!

Here are a few simple tips to follow in bringing the generations together:

Keep It simple. Alzheimer's disease is difficult for adults to understand, much less children. Use metaphors, symbols, and easy-to-understand analogies when explaining the disease. With teenagers, suggest ways in which they can become involved in caring for your loved one.

Keep it slow. Too much information can easily overwhelm young children. In this instance, less is more. Allow your children to integrate as much information as they can handle at their own pace. Allow your children to ask questions along the way.

Keep the fear to a minimum. Speak concretely about what a child can expect from a loved one with a memory disorder. With Alzheimer's disease, for example, a loved one is more likely to forget a younger child's name. Explain that there is no connection between forgetfulness and love.

Intergenerational Programs - The Tools for Family Connection

How do you foster a sense of togetherness when there is already so much to do? Perhaps your family, like so many others in today's society, suffers from a "generation gap." At Leeza's Place, we've found that the generations can often be brought together by involving them in activities they find mutually rewarding and enjoyable. Even families that are lucky enough not to have "issues" can benefit from group activities; they provide an enjoyable and rejuvenating break in the routine. We call these activities Intergenerational Programs, and they allow caregiving families to revel in the joys of togetherness—a togetherness that frequently transcends arguments, misunderstandings and distance. And that means a healthier, happier you, even as the demands caregiving continue.

At Leeza's Place, scrapbooking, journaling, stamping and Memory Television have become mainstays for helping caregivers and their families. Loved ones can participate; children can join in; and those of us who have never been "crafty" can enjoy these simple, yet emotionally and spiritually nourishing activities. These activities tap into each family member's innate creativity, and they can easily be adapted to your home setting. Let's take a closer look at them and see how you and your family can integrate them into your caregiving routine.

SCRAPBOOKING

Nathan (age 11): Sometimes when we'd go see J.G., I would feel worried and scared. But I never told anybody. I wish I had talked with my friends or my cousins or with my Mom. People can help you through things, even scary things. You don't want to keep it to yourself.

I wish I'd had more time with J.G. before she got sick. My friends have their grand moms and it makes me feel sad and sometimes mad. I feel worse for Pops than I do for me, though, because they were an awesome couple and they loved each other. I know J.G. was a good wife and I feel bad for Pops because I know he's been through a lot and to end up with something like this is painful. I hope Pops will take extra good care of himself because of all the stress.

I remember making scrapbook pages about J.G. and our family and our pets. When you do that it makes you feel better because you think of all the good times and what a happy person they used to be. I was so proud of my grand mom because she was so brave about Alzheimer's. When I look at scrapbook pictures of when she was younger I could tell she

was a person who owned up to who she was. You can see her
courage in the pictures.

Memories matter. Scrapbooking preserves these life treasures
on paper. Scrapbooks reflect how we lived, how we spent our time,
who we loved, and where we've been. We can record our own stories, from a simple memory of a night shared with friends to the
remarkable memory of a child's birth. Scrapbooking makes sure our
stories survive to share with future generations of our families.

As we sort through photographs with our loved ones and families, we also begin to sort through the new reality of Alzheimer's
disease, or whatever we may be up against. At a time when life is
increasingly out of control, photographs provide a tangible connection to our past, letting us feel a little safer and more comfortable.
Our loved ones can regain some power and dignity through the
process of scrapbooking as we pay attention to and honor these tangible records of their life stories.

Leeza: I flip through the pages of various scrapbooks, deeply
grateful for the warm feelings I get every time. With each pic-
ture, Mom comes alive and I keep a little bit of her close to
me. There's one picture of me at age five with a goofy flip in
my hair, around my ears. I remember asking Mom "What
were you thinking, fixing my hair like that?" She replied,
"Darlin', one day you're gonna look at this picture, remember
this conversation and smile at the very thought of that flippy
hair." She was right, I do.

If you can cut, tape and glue, you have all the skills needed for
scrapbooking. There's no wrong way to make your own scrapbook.
Once you have a general idea of what project you'd like to work

LEEZA'S SCRAPBOOK IDEA STARTERS

It's up to you to make certain your family legacy lives on. Jump-start the brainstorming your heritage pages by asking yourself these questions:

What are your parents' full names? Your grandparents'? How did they meet and fall in love? What were their religions? Where were they born?

Were you named for anyone in the family? What regional distinctions did you pick up? A southern drawl? A love for New England lobster rolls?

Which characters in your family always provide the drama? How would you describe them?

Who most influences your personality? For example, did you inherit your grandmother's passion for cats? Or your mother's love of flea markets?

What did your ancestors do for a living? What kind of house did they live in? Do you remember visiting any of them?

What world events influenced your parents or grandparents? If they're alive, ask them to describe the impact. Use a voice recorder so no detail is lost.

Is there a theme or event you want to make your scrapbook about? You can pick an occasion, a beloved person or pet, or begin the first of a series about your family story.

on, starting can be broken down into three easy steps: choosing an album, gathering supplies, and getting out your photos. Every photo a person takes or keeps is a type of self portrait, a "mirror with memory" reflecting back those moments and people that were special enough to be frozen in time. Collectively, these photographs make visible the ongoing stories of a person's life, and serve as a visual map of the past. Personal snapshots permanently record important daily moments and serve as natural bridges for accessing, exploring, and communicating about feelings and memories.

Sifting through a thousand random photographs might make you want to give up on scrapbooking altogether. If you want to do more than just get them into chronological order, consider sorting them into categories such as these:

- Family members. For example, pick out all the photographs of each child and put them in order chronologically.
- Holidays.
- Pets.
- Vacations.
- Sports events.

If you have digital photographs, you can print them out and use them just as easily as regular photographs. In fact, it's better not to risk damaging original photographs. Take your photos to be copied, or scan and print them.

Your scrapbook is more than just a conversation piece: it's a map of your life, your thoughts, your feelings, your memories. The act of creating these treasured pages, especially with your family members, can be therapeutic in ways you've never dreamed of. Assembling the pages triggers memories, prompts conversation and creates a bridge across which the generations can communicate. As a caregiver, your

ESSENTIAL SCRAPBOOKING TOOLS

Scissors. Find a pair with sharp, narrow points for fine cutting.

Paper Cutter. It's invaluable for cutting straight edges and measuring as you cut.

Crafts Knife. It's excellent for cutting out photo mats and for positioning small elements such as stickers.

Double-Sided Tape. It comes in different widths in handy dispensers that make it easy to use.

Glue Sticks. They make it simple to control the amount of adhesive you apply.

Photo Splits. Apply these small squares just as you would double-sided tape, then peel off the backing to expose the sticky side.

Journaling Pens. Make sure they're pigment or permanent ink, acid free, light fast, waterproof, and non-bleeding.

Ruler. Pick one with a metal edge to measure paper and use with a crafts knife.

Paper Punches. Use them to make all sorts of shapes, from hearts to hexagons.

world becomes a little easier to navigate with every feeling expressed, every memory shared, each moment spent in peace with your family. And when you scrapbook, you're left with a lasting souvenir!

For much more on scrapbooking, please refer to the Resources section at the end of this book.

FIVE STEPS FOR MAKING A SCRAPBOOK PAGE

1. Sort through your photos and chose those that document a favorite story or event. There's no magic number – sometimes you'll need only one photo, other times you'll need a dozen.

2. Go shopping! Take your photos with you so you can pick out papers and embellishments that will compliment them.

3. Borrow a page design. Craft magazines and scrapbooking books are filled with terrific design ideas. When rendered in different colors, and with your photos, the pages will have a look that's all your own.

4. Choose a title for the page and jot down a few notes for your journaling.

5. Play! Move around the elements on the page. Don't adhere anything permanently until the artist within you is completely satisfied.

JOURNALING

Everyone can write a journal. Journaling gives family members a private space to express difficult feelings, and a journal can become a quiet oasis away from the busy world of caregiving. When we journal, we can explore our inner thoughts and feelings without pressure and fear of reproach from others. We can talk about the grief, anger, frustration, and joy of caregiving without censoring our words. A journal can become a close friend during times of great change and stress. Anne Frank was so comforted by hers that she gave it a name: Kitty.

The simple act of putting our thoughts and feelings on paper can become a powerful means of facilitating family togetherness. As we "talk" with our journal, we often find the words we need to communicate with our family members about our deepest emotions. And, as we'll see later in this chapter, your family's journal pages can form the foundation of the "script" for your family's own "Memory Television." There's nothing to lose when you journal, and so much to gain. Taking the time to write is a wonderful first step to self-care and self-awareness. It's a great way to let your feelings flow, which frees more energy for the tasks of caregiving. Each sentence you write, either for yourself or with a family member, becomes another step towards discovering the magic of being truly energized.

STAMPING

Stamping, which is using stamps to put interesting designs on paper and cards, is a fascinating, creative and stress-free way to connect with friends and family. Stamping used to be mainly for serious "crafters", but in recent years it has become a broadly popular activity, especially as a means for making greeting cards. Stamps are available at most craft stores and stationery supply centers and there are many magazines and websites devoted entirely to stamping. We've come a long way since the days of simple construction paper; now, unusual papers and elegant materials are available to even the casual stamper. Is it hard? Not at all! Just push and stamp to create lasting mementoes.

Julie, one of our Leeza's Place clients, has been her grandmoth-

JOURNALING IN A NUTSHELL

The Basics. When journaling, think of the who/what/where/ when and why of the story you're telling. Set aside ideas about what your journal "should" be. This is a space where expectations and judgments can disappear and you don't need to make something beautiful or profound.

Throw Away the Rules! You don't have to anything in your journal, and that includes writing in complete sentences, using both sides of a page, or writing in the lines. Do what inspires you to write and what feels good.

Photo Captions. Add a caption for each photo or identify a group of photos. It can be as simple as the location where the photo was taken, the full name of the person pictured, or the date when the event took place.

Bulleted List. Make a list of the items you took on a camping trip, your dog's favorite toys, or the dishes served at a dinner party you threw.

Stories. These are the treasured memories passed down from generation to generation. They don't have to be long. Use specific details to convey information that photos can't. Describe the setting, what people wore, how foods tasted, the sounds in the background, or the way you felt at the time the picture was taken.

Poems, Quotes and Lyrics. Whether they're your own or were written by someone else, these can enhance a page with special sentiment. For ideas, head to the library reference section or do an internet search based on a particular theme, such as friendship or parenthood.

Handwritten or Typed. Some people avoid journaling because they feel their handwriting is messy or difficult to read. That's a shame! You can print journal entries from a computer for a neat presentation. Alphabet stencils, stickers and rub-on letters can add to your layouts. But it's important to include your own handwriting on a page, even if it's just a signature or a date written longhand. It's unique to you and will communicate its own message for generations to come.

er's caregiver for almost ten years. She told us that her two young children were unsure of how to relate to an older person, and her disease frightened them at first. Someone suggested spending an evening together making cards with stamps. Julie remembers, "I was not into the idea because I am not a very creative person. But I needed to try something to bring Grandma into the scene that wasn't scary for the little ones. As it turned out, they loved it! Grandma really got into it, and to my surprise, so did I. Now we have six boxes of stamps and a regular stamping night. Grandma is pretty disabled, but she sits with us and smiles at the things the kids come up with. The kids and I love making cards to acknowledge family milestones, holidays, or 'just because.' Best of all, the moments we spend together in harmony give me a sense of strength and peace that lasts long after our little workshop session has finished. There's more calm at home and let me tell you, as a parent that goes a long way!"

Julie was pleasantly surprised by how easy it was to begin stamping, and you may be, too. You can pick out a few nice papers and one or two stamps to begin with, and then buy more elaborate supplies as desired. Try unusual ink colors, or layering with translucent papers for a different effect. Your loved one can make his or her own card, or may enjoy working with someone. Find paper with rough grain or embossed patterns and let them feel the various textures as a way to involve them more deeply in the activity. For more about stamping, please refer to the Resources section at the end of this book.

MEMORY TELEVISION™: A VIDEO STARRING YOU AND YOUR LOVED ONES

Everyone has a story, and our stories are interwoven with those of our family and friends. Sharing our family history with others brings connection and deep relief for those who are losing precious memories and for their caregivers as well. By recording the stories of our lives on video or DVD, we are able to ensure that others will witness them and that we will not be forgotten. At Leeza's Place we call this Leeza's Memory Television™, and you can do it at home.

Families are amazed at how much fun it is, and how deeply rewarding it can be, to record their personal stories. Many family members hear something they never knew, or learn something new, through this process. One Leeza's Place visitor was stunned to see a tear roll down her husband's cheek during filming as he recalled the death of his infant sister many years before. "I never realized he was so affected by that experience," she recalls. "We've been married 51 years and this is the first time he's really talked about her."

Often, loved ones are moved by hearing how much they mean to their family and friends. Elizabeth, a widow and Alzheimer's disease patient, resented being moved to her daughter's house, though she was incapable of remaining in her own apartment any longer. She was especially irritable around Thomas, her son-in-law, even as he worked hard to help her feel welcome in their home. During the taping of their family video, Thomas spoke into the camera and said that Elizabeth's husband had meant a great deal to him. He also knew how much her husband had meant to Elizabeth, and how much she missed him, and so he hoped to be the man in her life now that her spouse was gone. After watching the film, Elizabeth returned to Leeza's Place a changed woman. She said, "Watching my son-in-law in that movie made me realize that I am at their house for a reason. My husband is gone but Thomas wants to be that strength for me now." The experience transformed her resentment and helped her feel less of a burden to her family—which in turn made the family feel more at ease. Here's how you and your family can make video memories at home:

Step 1: Scriptwriting.

You may want your recording to be an epic, but if you want to limit its length, it helps to write a script. Don't worry; you don't need stage directions and lines of dialogue! Memories are all you need. Reading books and studying a family tree may provide facts and names, but not the real character of a family. It's the personal stories of daily life that vividly illustrate where we've come from, and perhaps where we're heading. These "best selling" stories come from those we love: elders, caregivers and children. They can make us laugh or cry, provide wisdom and give insight. Most importantly, capturing our story and the stories of our loved ones allows us to heal and be accepting of loss.

Bring your family together. Give everyone an opportunity to remember the good times and accomplishments they have experienced, and jot them down. This will help ensure that when the "director" yells "Action" you won't forget anything. That's it! Your script is ready to shoot.

Step 2: Set Design

Although some people are satisfied with a simple backdrop such as their family room, many like to create a special environment for their video. For Leeza's Memory Television we use photographs, in addition to scrapbooks and family keepsakes, to form the visual background for each family's unique video.

Step 3: Action!

Using your script and backdrop, let the memories flow. Future generations will treasure the details of the past, and existing generations will feel enriched by details of the lives of those they love.

Connecting As A Family - The Payoff

"My sweet boys…" Troy remembers his visit with his grandmother at the nursing home, when she showed that the connection of family love can be stronger even than the power of progressive memory loss. "At just 10 years old I learned a lesson that has not left me ever since and never will. The presence of a person is not their physical being; it's their energy, their soul, their inner being. No matter what happens to them, whether they lose their memory or lose their life, they really didn't lose anything. As long as they have touched the hearts of their loved ones, and the people on this earth still care for them and still love them, they will never leave. J.G. is here with us right now, and so is every other person with this disease. If it feels like they are gone, just listen: they're inside of you, all around you, listening to what you have to say. So speak up and talk to them, and talk to your other loved ones. The more connected you feel to your family, the stronger you'll feel."

Caregiving can become the means by which you and your family can revel in each other's strength and companionship. Taking the time to enjoy creative activities as a family will help free everyone's mind, heart and spirit for the road ahead. And you, the caregiver, will feel a palpable sense of connection with your loved ones that will give you the strength to carry on. With those around you working together, communicating and enjoying each other's company, your anxiety will decrease. Because you feel a greater sense of support, you'll be less prone to fall into the self-punishing realm of guilt. You'll be less burdened physically and emotionally. As a result, you will enjoy greater energy that will improve the quality of the life of the loved on in your care – and in your own life, too.

CHAPTER 11

Caregiving as a
Spiritual Practice

*L**eeza: You have sole custody of your life, so step up and own it. This usually means you have to reinvent yourself constantly. You have to stretch and bend, or you will break.*

Leeza and her family found that caring for Jean was a constant struggle to remain flexible, to be open to seeing her, themselves and the world in a fresh way from moment to moment. They found, as many caregivers do, that a vital way to hold onto their own being was to let go of Jean as they had known her and the accept the inevitability of their loss.

When a loved one dies, we normally grieve and take refuge in the memories we have of him. It is how we all find the capacity to continue on with our own lives. It is a completely different challenge, however, when a loved one is still physically alive but is losing (or has lost) his intellectual and emotional moorings. How do you go on when a loved one is no longer present in mind but still present in body?

"The hard thing about losing Jean to Alzheimer's over the years was that there was no closure," Carlos, Sr. recalls. "As Jean got worse, all the familiar chapters of our lives came to a close. But with time I found that as those chapters ended, new ones opened." It is these new chapters, this new life with your loved one, which you must embrace in order to cope with the emotional turmoil brought about by the disease and with the sad fact that you cannot hope for no improvement in your loved one's life. For example, your loved one may no longer recognize you or he may recognize the sound of your voice but not know you by your name or understand the relationship you share. But he may now enjoy it when you sing for him or perhaps when you simply hold his hand and listen to music together. The complicated nature of a relationship based on shared memories quite often gives way to the simple touch and feel of experiencing the present moment.

With memory loss disorders, there is no comfort to be found in hoping for future recovery or improvement. If we don't grieve for what we have lost, we can't experience what we have now. Consider the Tibetan spiritual training philosophy that instructs one to "abandon all hope of fruition." Rather than encourage despair, this adage is meant to give its practitioners strength by *freeing them* from hope, specifically the hope of receiving rewards for one's labors. By letting go of the hope of improvement, we are able to enter more fully into the work of the moment and the inherent joy of a life lived in the present, rather than looking ahead to something better "out there." To abandon hope does not mean to give up. It just means to let go: to let go of the hope that your acts of compassion will help the person regain his memory. *Caregiving is a practice of the present tense.*

You can grieve for the life that was and for the one that will not be. Grieve that your mom doesn't know she is at your son's baseball game. Grieve that your once dapper dad no longer knows how to tie his tie. Grieve that your librarian wife can no longer read a book. Grieve for all of these losses and more, and then let them go. It is only by letting go of the person that was that you can discover the person that is and bring peace to yourself.

This is true not just regarding the loved one you are caring for, but for your own life as well. In the end, life isn't about choosing what happens to us; we only get to choose how to respond to it. Caregiving is a long and arduous journey that requires great reserves of strength, humor, willingness and a commitment not be held prisoner by expectations of "what should be." There are no "shoulds" in caregiving; there is only "what is."

Finding Meaning In Your Life

Billy Graham once said, "I do not believe mere suffering teaches us. If that were so, the whole world would be wise!" Whether you believe that suffering is God's way of creating better people or that suffering is a random, meaningless, but unavoidable part of life, what is ultimately important is how we find the meaning in our lives despite the suffering. How can we make hardship, grief, or loss meaningful? How can we use the pain to transform our lives and find greater peace? As the great Jewish rabbi David Wolpe wrote, "We grow not by solving riddles but by creating meaning."

When pain and suffering become overwhelming, we try nearly anything to find relief. We struggle to come up with new strategies to minimize the potential of getting hurt. But when these strategies no longer work, our only option is to face our pain. When we are willing to stop running from what is too difficult, our pain lessens. We begin to recognize some of the mistaken beliefs we have operated under, such as, "If I do everything right, I will be safe and comfortable." As we discussed previously, we recognize some of the defenses we have constructed to avoid pain, such as denial and anger, and realize that they are actually increasing our pain. We learn that the difficulties faced on the caregiving journey aren't obstacles to living a full life; on the contrary, the difficulties we face can help us to truly appreciate and embrace our lives.

Carlos, Sr.'s O2 for Caregivers

KEEPING IT POSITIVE

From milking cows as a kid to running for governor as an adult, I always gained a sense of satisfaction from tackling the task at hand; I always retained my spirit. Then I experienced caregiving. For the first time in my life, I began to feel irritable, hopeless and helpless. It's vital to avoid succumbing to these emotions. If you feel blue, irritable and/or helpless:

- Find a support group and connect with people.
- Find a psychologist, a social worker or a counselor to really gauge "how blue is blue."
- Look learning opportunities in all challenging or negative events.
- If one door is closed, seek another open door to step through.

Accepting the Pain

Too often, we mistakenly believe that the cause of our suffering lies outside ourselves; that there is something or someone external to us creating our discomfort. But the cause of our pain is really *resistance itself*. It's painful to fight what we cannot change. While grief is a natural response to loss, the burning pain of resistance is unnecessary. In struggling against our loved one's diagnosis, against the reality of the disease, and by giving in to the urge to feel bad about ourselves, we increase our own suffering.

It's easy to understand this concept if we consider our natural fear of physical pain. A five year-old girl was very sick and was taken to the doctor's office so that a drop of blood could be drawn from her finger for testing. The child was terribly frightened; she screamed and fought all the way to the doctor's office and during the entire time in the waiting room. But, in the actual moment of the pin prick, the girl felt only a second of mild pain—nothing as painful as her fear and struggle to avoid it. In the end, it was really the child's struggle to avoid pain that caused her the greatest suffering.

We are afraid to suffer, so naturally we try to avoid it. This resistance to the unchangeable drains us of physical and emotional energy: we wake up tired no matter how much sleep we've gotten the night before. We dread the day, wanting only to look ahead to a point when things might be different, or look back and reminisce about easier times. We feel weak, disempowered by circumstance. But when we stop fighting the pain and accept what cannot be changed, when we allow our tragedies to exist without trying to escape from them, we can find renewed energy and make peace with our circumstances, however unpleasant. This isn't to say one should "give up" or be passive. Acceptance is about *embracing* those things that we cannot change and, more importantly, about choosing to experience *all* of life —not just what we want to experience.

The stress and pain of caregiving sometimes lead to what some call "a dark night of the soul," a time of despair when all seems terribly overwhelming and we must decide if we will answer life's call, a call to change our behavior in order to fulfill a purpose higher than our own comfort. But this bottommost point presents the opportunity for us to be transformed into more powerful, self-aware and capable people. When our resistance to reality fades, we begin to experience it for what it is and not what we want it to be. We stop wasting energy in a fruitless attempt to avoid pain, freeing up that energy for ourselves. Importantly, by facing the bad, we reveal the good within ourselves, the power we are frequently unaware of. We can banish the guilt that holds us back, the fear that makes us want to hide. The psychiatrist and author M. Scott Peck understood this when he wrote, "…our finest moments are most likely to occur when we are feeling deeply uncomfortable, unhappy, or unfulfilled. For it is only in such moments, propelled by our discomfort, that we are likely to step out of our ruts and start searching for different ways or truer answers." We cannot find the wisdom, cannot be "propelled by our discomfort" when we are resisting. We must first choose acceptance.

> *Leeza: When Mom began to succumb to the Alzheimer's disease I resisted the reality of it. But she ultimately gave us such a gift –by recognizing her disease and forcing us to deal with it. Her courageous rejection of denial ultimately freed her and the family as well.*

Caregiving presents an opportunity to learn acceptance, to live in the present moment and let go of what we can't control. It's an opportunity to stop wasting our precious energy by resisting reality and instead embrace life fully, with all its pains and joys. We each have a choice. Will we continue to fight, creating more pain for ourselves, or will we accept life on life's terms and really live?

For a caregiver to succeed and even thrive under the duress of caring for a loved one with memory loss, she must become a kind of soldier, what those who practice Buddhism call a "warrior of compassion." Rather than be beaten down by what feels like the war the disease is waging with your loved one, volunteer to "join the action". Not as a soldier fighting the disease head to head, but rather, as a compassionate medic under fire, caring for the wounded, making the fallen as comfortable as possible as the battle rages on.

Alan, one of our clients, dramatically illustrates the transformative effects of caregiving that he experienced when he was forced to deal with his father, who had been battling memory loss for years. He remembers the choice he ultimately came up against: to embrace his life or to turn away from the pain. "I remember how I fought to find meaning in Dad's suffering, and my own. I read every book on spirituality I could find, from Shamanism to Christianity to Buddhism. Each of them called for people to help alleviate suffering in the world. Examining my own life, I realized that I had *caused* pain, to myself and to others. My father's heartbreaking, gradual death reminded me daily of my own life and my own mortality. I didn't want to continue along as I had. I had to really decide what kind of person I wanted to be, and ultimately I learned to open up my heart. In the process of remaining close to my dad and letting the pain in, I found real meaning for the first time. Before, I had always chosen to avoid the bigger, more painful parts of life. By staying with my pain, with all the fears that came along as well, I could also really feel the life and joy which had been so elusive in the past. By trusting in life, and braving the pain, I think we discover something greater than fear, greater than pain, something which is truly who and what we are: eternal."

Like Alan, when we make the decision to actively choose what life has irrevocably chosen for us, we exercise our power. A choice like this may be the most difficult one we will ever face. But it can save us. It allows us to stop running and to begin confronting life, which in turn frees up untold amounts of energy: energy needed for the marathon of providing care to a loved one with a degenerative memory disorder, energy needed to live fulfilling lives of our own.

> *Leeza: Time passes so quickly and the person you love will slip away whether you are ready to face it or not. Refusing to accept the disease, or fighting against its progression, saps you of energy and of meaning in your life. By facing my mother's illness and being able to tell her story, we've brought meaning and hope back into our family. Rather than fighting the truth of her disease, we've been able to turn that energy into the positive hope that is Leeza's Place—to make something meaningful and beautiful out of our suffering.*

Taking on the care of a loved one is an opportunity to open the heart's capacity to live fully, even in the midst of enormous loss. As examples, watching our loved ones suffer memory loss can open our eyes to some rather unpleasant aspects of our own lives and natures: that we haven't made authentic personal connections with others, including our families; that we don't know ourselves very well; that we have an unrealistic view of our life and our world. This process of examining ourselves is known as a "breaking open": a time when our guards have been let down. It is when we are in this vulnerable space that we have an opportunity to find real meaning in our lives.

How do you find meaning for yourself during this challenging and painful time? First, recognize that the search for meaning, this "breaking open" is an important opportunity, a "head start" towards greater self awareness and personal growth. It's important to seize this opportunity and make the most of it.

Second, it helps to seek out a *spiritual companion*, a family member or someone else who is close to you and with whom you can share your thoughts. You may wish to seek out others who have more experience with caregiving, such as religious advisors or older people. You might find a support group for people facing the same challenges as you. Perhaps you will find it especially meaningful to share your journey with someone much younger than you, for the fresh perspective they bring.

Serious illness, either our own or another person's, often pushes us to reevaluate our priorities and values and can force us to rethink what really matters to us. Often, we discover that what matters most are our relationships with ourselves, with others, and with the world around us. Our grief for our loved one can help strip us of superficial relationships, dreams and desires, and leave us with genuine connectedness. The "practice" of caring for our loved ones is an opportunity to learn and grow – not *despite* the challenges and troubles, but *because* of them.

The Dalai Lama is joyful as he comforts the sick and the impoverished. Gandhi was joyful as he walked mile after mile in protest of injustice and fasted for the right to be considered an equal. Martin Luther King was vibrant with joy, though his life was under constant threat. Why were these people able to feel joy in the midst of such suffering? Because they did not dwell in suffering. They put themselves in the middle of their lives with a full heart. Such a way of life gives one meaning and allows one to feel fully alive. Joy is not the fleeting satisfaction of material happiness; it's not a life of ease. Joy is finding meaning and wisdom. For you, the caregiver, such a life awaits you if you embrace the challenges of caregiving and forge ahead.

Living the Why of Caregiving

Caregiving for a loved one with a degenerative memory disorder requires countless physical, emotional, and social sacrifices. For this reason, we can't allow it to cause a loss of meaning in our lives as well. We must have meaning in our tasks and in our lives because meaning is the fuel of life, it's what keep us going. Develop your reason to keep going into a "caregiver credo" and live by it. Your credo could be a simple as, *"I commit to making sure that I use this caregiving experience to grow, become wiser, stronger, and to let go of my loved one day by day as I honor what she was and what she is now."*

A credo like this should be written down and placed in a variety of locations around the home where it can be seen throughout the day. This way, you reinforce it with the passage of time, and in so doing, transform it into a way of life. Other rituals can be practiced that reinforce your credo. They don't have to be complicated or formalized. Your rituals could begin every morning, when you go into the room to wash your loved one. With each dip of the washcloth into warm water, you can think to yourself, "I am dipping this cloth in the water that washes off the night and brings on the day. With this cloth I am entering this present moment." As you use the cloth to wash the various parts of your loved one's body you can think, "I honor your hands, which once built furniture, wrote books, built houses, dug ditches, did accounting, wrote computer code..." For the legs, it could be to honor the dancing, the walking, and all the places this person has traveled in life. You can say these things out loud, making each body part you touch another opportunity to bring connection and dignity to yourself and to the person for whom you are caring. Don't worry that it might seem as though you are having a one-way conversation with your loved one. Anyone who has been caregiving for a while knows that it is not required that a dialogue be verbal. The important point is that you are hearing the words and they are having a cumulative effect on *you*.

Part of the day's rituals can also be focused on entering the present moment of where your loved one is now. They can still feel sensation, so walk them barefoot on the grass or on the beach or in the muddy marsh. Put different shapes in their hands: sea shells, rocks rough and smooth, moss, grass, bark, little cars and toys, the hand or foot of a baby, a cat or puppy or anything else you have on hand.

Music is a proven way for those with degenerative memory disorders to connect in the present moment. So if you are a musician, play. If you have friends that play, invite them over. If your loved one is able, bring him to concerts. Or, find out when local schools have performances. Doing these things will help your loved one feel less isolated, and just as importantly, it will keep *you* from becoming too isolated. People will begin to recognize you. They will begin to look for you and your loved one. Your loved one will have a new place of importance to be and so will you.

Cammy: We tried hard to keep my son, Blake, age 7, involved with his grandmother Jean as much as possible. Blake just naturally seemed to find the good in all the sadness around us, as you can see from my talks with him while Jean was in hospice and when she passed away:

At J.G.'s bedside...
  Blake: J.G. knows it's me when I touch her.
  Me: Do you think she can feel you hold her hand?
  Blake: She can feel me touch her heart.

After visiting with J.G....
  Blake: Mama, will you write down everything for me in case you get sick like J.G.? I want to always be able to communicate with you.
  Me: (pulling off the road in tears) I promise baby. I will write as much as I can and it will still never be enough.
  Blake: (wipes my tears with his little hand) But you al-

ways say a heart doesn't forget, so I will know you forever. Even if you can't talk, I'll still know you.

After J.G. died...

Blake: (seeing two wispy clouds that do look like the letters "J" and "G" and then are scattered in the air). Look Mom, there's J.G. in the clouds! J.G. is in the wind now and she can go anywhere she wants.

At J.G.'s gravesite...

Me: Blake, it's not respectful to dance on someone's grave. Stop it!

Blake: But J.G. loved to dance. You should dance with me.

Linda, one of our guests at Leeza's Place, experienced a profound moment of personal and spiritual growth from observing the simplest of rituals: watching her father eat. "My father moved in with my husband, my two children, and me two months before his diagnosis of Alzheimer's disease," she recalls. "I was sure I could manage through will power alone. Then I realized this wasn't going to go away; there was no cure. That realization was the hardest." Linda grew weary as the illness dragged on for years. Knowing her father would never be well again, it seemed like a terrible and pointless battle to fight through each day just waiting for the inevitable. "It was so painful to watch his slow descent into death. I began to question not just my own efforts but ultimately the meaning of life in general."

Linda found herself getting more and more tired in a way that went beyond the physical. "I finally realized I had to actively find meaning in what I was doing or find someplace else for my father. I didn't want to send him away, but I knew I was going to get sick myself unless something changed." And it was when Linda was at this low point that she had a life changing moment of self discovery. "I was sitting with him at the table. He had started to eat meals with his fingers, which had begun to disgust me. I wanted to stop him, to get up and leave, but I stayed. I just sat there and let him be and watched him. And it struck me: how much I loved him, even as I hated the sickness that was taking over. Something in me suddenly relaxed. I didn't understand it right away, but something was released and I felt such a clear energy. I started to cry there at the table with my dad. I had been pushing and pulling against this disease from the start, fighting what was beyond my control. It was only when I opened myself up to this man as he was and to the pain as it was, that real love and acceptance could return."

Though Linda's caregiving responsibilities are no less arduous, her change of viewpoint has provided real relief to her life and spirit. "I am finding energy instead of despair," she declares, "even though there is still so much sadness. I'm learning to relate to my father in his changing state, and even learning how to relate to my husband and children better as well. I look back at who I was before I became this caregiver, and though I miss the feeling of control and security I used to have, I am grateful for the person I've become. I feel a level of love and connection that wasn't there before."

Linda has learned to alternate between honoring the past and engaging with the present. That means staying with activities that bring a sense of dignity and productivity to you and your loved one. When feelings come up that such things are fruitless, remember that this voice of despair represents the most tired part of you trying to be heard. Listen to it. Show this tired self compassion. Ask it to put its feet up and let it share its woes, for an hour. But then gently send it on its way, because the rest of the day is for living.

It's not easy to keep going in the face of a future that does not

Carlos, Sr.'s O2 for Caregivers

STAY CONNECTED TO YOUR OWN LIFE

As time went on caring for Jean, I began to lose interest in the things I used to have a passion for and my sense of isolation from the rest of the world began to grow. I found myself turning to alcohol to deal with these losses. Don't let this happen to you!

REMEMBER:

- Find your own personal passion: a hobby, a movie night... and try to make room for it.
- Attend a support group. It helps to hear how you aren't alone in your experiences.
- Set up a buddy system with a family member, friend or neighbor who expects to hear from you on a regular basis.
- Find a "breakfast club" of your own and make it a pleasant routine.
- Don't self-medicate! It does not help, it only compounds your inability to cope.
- See a professional. Find out if your loss of interest is due to treatable depression.

improve in the traditional way that we think about "improvement" and "progress." But this should not matter to you. The caregiving experience can be the work which allows us to realize our true power and ability to triumph over hardship and see what is good in life. Carlos, Sr. is a great example of that transformation. Since Jean's passing, he has continued going to support groups, and he still goes to breakfast with his old friends at their favorite dining spot in Irmo. He also does volunteer work at Lowman House, the residential setting that took such good care of his one and only Jean. Carlos became his own healer, and is today as committed to the ongoing work of healing himself as he was during Jean's decline. You can do the same.

Cammy: Several years ago while packing away Mom's things I found a little cigar box with all of her gloves inside. They were so tiny I could hardly fit my hand into them (funny, I remember thinking her hands had always seemed so large, but they were really quite petite). For me, the gloves brought back memories of her sliding them on to leave the house for an event with Dad. When I was a girl I used to love to watch her get ready and transform herself from Mom to Princess. She was incredibly beautiful.

When I wrote this poem, Mom was at the nursing home but she could still sometimes curl her fingers around mine when I went to hold her hand. I don't know why I waited until this past Christmas to give a copy of this poem along with a pair of her gloves to Carl and Leez. Maybe it was because Mom hadn't been able to curl her fingers around my hand in so long; maybe some part of me knew we would never feel her hands squeeze ours again. I'm crying again as I write this. Anyway, I guess you never really want to let go of your mother's hand. It's not really written very well, but it's how I feel about Mom:

Worn by hands that held me often,
Soothed my fevered brow,
Administered care to cuts and bruises,
Wiped away tears, Cooked all my favorite meals,
Sewed buttons and hems,
Flipped through pages of storybooks,
Gardened, Painted,
and were often,
Clenched with worry for me.
The hands that wore these gloves
shook hands with dignitaries, smoked too many cigarettes,
often held a bourbon and ginger,
and struggled in vain to write a story
she never fully understood.
Hands that favored larger jewels,
but never the indulgence of a manicure.
The woman who wore these gloves
belonged to an era that I will never know.
She often wore these gloves
with her hair piled high into a platinum masterpiece
secured with a tiara.
These gloves were worn by hands
that I will forever wish to hold again.
These gloves belonged to my mother,
Gloria Jean Dyson Gibbons
Southern Belle, Steel Magnolia

Finding Meaning in Caregiving - The Payoff

"I know firsthand that the caregiving experience can be the thing that allows you to realize your ability to triumph over hardship and see what's good in life," Carlos, Sr. declares.

Carlos has come a long way for the exhausted husband whose physical and emotional health were so challenged during his darkest hours with Jean's illness. "When I was in my darkest hours, I couldn't have imagined that there would be a time when I would view myself as a stronger and more capable person because of this experience. But that's just what happened." Like Alan and Linda from Leeza's Place, and the entire Gibbons family, you can use the experience of caregiving to understand and celebrate the many dimensions your life can encompass. By remaining open to the pain and staying with the questions that arise, you will come to realize that you are a powerful person. The constant strain of resistance will fade away as you accept the difficulties – and the potential joys – of your caregiving role. By taking your oxygen first, you'll find that your spirit is ready to face whatever awaits you on the road ahead.

Congratulations! You can now reap the benefits of the Three E's: Education, Empowerment and Energy. You are now more educated about the challenges facing your loved one and yourself. You have moved beyond merely educating yourself and are connecting with your physical self and with your own emotions. And of course, you are experiencing the increased physical and mental energy that comes with reducing your stress and anxiety. You now embrace a fundamental truth of caregiving: that effective caregiving begins by taking care of your own mind, body and spirit. You have learned that you deserve a full life and you can experience great joy, even while giving care to a loved one with a memory loss disorder. With this renewed energy, you now have the ability to rise to any occasion and can accomplish anything you believe in, both in caregiving and in every other aspect of your life.

Afterword

GOODBYE TO JEAN

A mother's love is a sturdy thing. It survives most everything in its path. It endures immeasurable heartache, faces overwhelming fears, creates magic and miracles, and challenges all enemies. A mother's love can comfort and soothe, correct and scold, guide and let go all with one look. It is steady and constant - omnipresent and solid.

Yes, a mother's love is a sturdy thing, but life is ultimately not. Children, no matter how old, have an irrational belief that their moms will last forever. We can't quite figure out who we are without the one who gave us life to define us. When mothers die, it leaves the ones left behind desperate to find that true north on the compass.

But a mother's love is sturdy. It doesn't collapse under the grief of loss. It lasts beyond the expiration of the earthly vessel that kissed boo-boos and tucked us in at night. A mother's love is deposited into the hearts of those she loved and there it grows and lives forever. It is sturdy enough to prop us up and remind us of the courage she taught us. Sturdy enough to create a veil of peace until we can find serenity on our own.

My mom has been emancipated from the prison of confusion that kept her hostage for a decade. Her love is surely sturdy enough for me to climb onto its wake of protection and stay there while we make sense of her suffering and her courageous battle against Alzheimer's disease. Her death was the answer to the prayers my Dad, brother and sister and I have whispered and spoken aloud for some time. Death, of course, is not on our clock and yet there is perfection in the timing of the universe. Gloria Jean Dyson Gibbons left a legacy of love and change that is powerful and beautiful.

At her urging, we shared her diagnosis and her story of truth and strength as a lifeline to others who were afraid and who felt alone. She asked me to promise to tell her story, and I continue to try. Our family started the Leeza Gibbons Memory Foundation as a love letter to my Mom and all the moms who know that love is love and a heart never forgets. We believe that those who are forgetting should not be forgotten and that no caregiver should ever be alone. And so we began to open Leeza's Place as an oasis for those families who know chronic disease of any kind. My mother's door was always open. She always had the coffee on and time for a conversation. It's that way at Leeza's Place. Like love, our support is free and is offered without conditions. I remember many conversations with my mother where she made it clear that she didn't want there to be shame surrounding her diagnosis. So we proudly embrace her spirit and celebrate her life.

They say the soul has an agenda. If that's true then my mom has checked this lifetime off the list! She has been the inspiration for so much healing and so much help that has been offered in her name. In South Carolina, we get amazing storms. Mom loved them. She related to the change in the atmosphere and always saw it as a chance at a new beginning. Like the storms she loved, she was outspoken and fearless and yet vulnerable and ready for a good downpour of emotion. Her dreams were simple. To love her family the best way she knew how and to find her true self along the way. She used to say she was a strong southern woman, a steel magnolia, and that God gave her such broad shoulders for a reason. It was to carry a dream of change. Mom, now that you have placed it down, Cammy, Carlos, Anne Marie and I will pick it up and carry it effortlessly and gracefully because we are supported by your sturdy love. My children and their children will keep the story vital and keep the flame burning brightly.

On the day Mom died, Daddy kissed his wife of 55 years good-bye. He said it was hard to let go of her and yet he too was relieved for her release. To those who have loved her and loved me or my family, I feel your support and your presence. We feel the collective blanket you are offering and we will wrap ourselves up in it and feel safe. Our family thanks you for your prayers, thoughts and outpouring of love.

Like millions of other families who bravely battle this insidious disease, we are dedicated to creating a world where memory loss no longer threatens. Through our work at Leeza's Place we are blessed to have created a nationwide caregiver community that has become better educated, and more empowered and energized to face their struggles. It is a beautiful legacy to our Mom, Dad's wife, Gloria Jean Dyson Gibbons.

—*Leeza*

She battled bravely for a decade while her mind was held hostage by Alzheimer's disease and slowly Gloria Jean Gibbons began to fade away, memory by memory. She was released from her fight on Thursday, May 22, 2008 when she passed away at the age of 72. Jean's insistence that her family tell her story was the inspiration for the Leeza Gibbons Memory Foundation and today Leeza's Place is her living legacy. Jean leaves behind Carlos, her husband of 55 years, their three children, Carlos, Jr., Leeza and Cammy, Carlos Jr.'s wife, Anne Marie, and six grandchildren, Lexi, Troy, Nathan, Taylor, Kelly and Blake.

Caregiver Resources

The following provides some of the many resources you can turn to for support, information and encouragement during your time giving care to your loved one.

General Alzheimer's disease Information and Resources

ADEAR (Alzheimer's Disease Education & Referral Center)
National Institute on Aging
31 Center Drive, MSC 2292
Building 31, Room 5C27
Bethesda, MD 20892
Phone: (301) 496-1752
Fax: (301) 496-1072
Website: http://www.nia.nih.gov/Alzheimers/AlzheimersInformation/GeneralInfo/
Current, comprehensive Information on Alzheimer's disease research, information, and resources from the National Institute on Aging.

Alzheimer's Association
225 N. Michigan Ave., 17th Floor
Chicago, IL 60601-7633
Phone and 24/7 helpline: (800) 272-3900
Website: http://www.alz.org
A national organization focusing on Alzheimer's disease care, support, information and research; its website includes a multilingual resources and search function.

Alzheimer's Foundation of America

322 8th Ave., 6th Floor

New York, NY 10001

Phone: (866) 232-8484

Website: http://www.alzfdn.org/

Provides care and services to individuals confronting dementia, their caregivers and their families.

The Alzheimer's Store

Phone: (800) 752-3238

Website: http://www.alzstore.com/

Products and services for those caring for someone with Alzheimer's disease.

Mayo Clinic.com

Website: http://www.mayoclinic.com/health/alzheimers/AZ99999

Information on Alzheimer's disease and other memory loss disorders, treatment, caregiving and helping young people understand these diseases.

National Institutes of Health Senior Health-Alzheimer's Disease

Website: http://nihseniorhealth.gov/alzheimersdisease/toc.html

A website about Alzheimer's disease for computer savvy seniors. for computer savvy seniors.

Regional Alzheimer's Resources

**Joseph and Kathleen Bryan Alzheimer's Disease
Research Center**
Duke University School of Medicine
2200 W. Main Street, Suite A200
Box 3503 DUMC
Durham, NC 27705
Phone: (919) 684-3633
Website: http://adrc.mc.duke.edu/
A clinical and basic science center dedicated to the highest
level care for patients and families affected by Alzheimer's disease
and other memory disorders.

University of Virginia
Department of Neurology
Memory Disorders Clinic
P.O. Box 800394
Charlottesville, VA 22908
Phone: (800) 251-3627
Website: http://www.healthsystem.virginia.edu/internet/neurol
ogy/what_we_treat/alzheimers/index.cfm
Dedicated to helping people cope with challenges brought on
by impaired memory and related complications.

Research Centers

**University of California San Francisco Memory and
Aging Center**
350 Parnassus Avenue, Suite 905

San Francisco, California 94117

(415) 476-6880

http://memory.ucsf.edu/

The Memory and Aging Center strives to provide the highest quality of care for individuals with cognitive problems, conduct research on the causes and cures for degenerative brain diseases, and educate health professionals, patients and their families.

Alzheimer's Disease Research Centers of California

http://www.cdph.ca.gov/programs/alzheimers/

Provides diagnostic and treatment services, education and support and promotes enhanced training of health care professionals, and supports research to discover the cause of and cure for Alzheimer's disease at ten locations in northern and southern California.

Southwestern Medical Center Alzheimer's disease Center

UT Southwestern Medical Center

James W. Aston Ambulatory Care Center

5323 Harry Hines Blvd.

Dallas, TX 75390

Phone: 214-648-3111

http://www.utsouthwestern.edu/utsw/cda/

The Alzheimer's disease Center at UT Southwestern is one of 32 centers funded by the National Institute on Aging to evaluate patients and to conduct scientific research into the cause(s) of Alzheimer's disease.

General Information on Aging

AREA AGENCY ON AGING

Every county in the United States has an agency that is responsible for distributing federal and local funds to support elderly citizens. These programs include Meals on Wheels, homemaker assistance, home care as an alternative to nursing home care, transportation, respite care, and other caregiver-related support programs. Find your local agency by looking in the white pages under "Area Agency on Aging" or go to http//www.eldercare.gov .

Focus on Healthy Aging
800 Connecticut Ave
Norwalk, CT 06854
Phone: (800) 829-9406
Website: http://www.focusonhealthyaging.com/
The Mount Sinai School of Medicine's monthly newsletter.

National Institute on Aging
Website: http://www.nia.nih.gov
Provides health and research information for seniors.

National Library of Medicine
8600 Rockville Pike
Bethesda, MD 20894
Phone: (888) 346-3656
Website: http://www.nlm.nih.gov/medlineplus/alzheimersdis
	ease.html
Provides links to numerous government agencies and nonprofit organizations and recent news on Alzheimer's disease.

healthfinder.gov
PO Box 133
Washington, D.C. 20013-1133
Website: http://www.healthfinder.gov
A resource for finding the best government and non-profit health services information.

Caregiver Support

Family Caregiver Alliance
180 Montgomery St, Ste 1100
San Francisco, CA 94104
Phone: (800) 445-8106
Fax: (415) 434-3508
Email: info@caregiver.org
Website: http://www.caregiver.org/
Provides information, education, services, research, advocacy and support to sustain the work of families nationwide caring for loved ones with chronic, disabling health conditions.

The Leeza Gibbons Memory Foundation
3050 Biscayne Blvd. Ste. 605
Miami, FL 33137
Telephone Number. (888) OK-Leeza
Website: www.leezasplace.org
Email: info@leezasplace.org

The flagship LGMF program is Leeza's Place, community centers affiliated with local health services programs where caregivers of individuals with memory and other disorders can find support, resources, guidance and information about giving care to their loved ones, their families and to themselves. You can find

Leeza's Place community centers at the following locations:

Leeza's Place at Olympia Medical Center
5901 West Olympic Blvd, Suite 300A
Los Angeles, California 90036
Tel 323-932-5414

Circle of Care Leeza's Place
5000 Van Nuys Boulevard, Suite 110
Sherman Oaks, CA 91403
Telephone: (818) 817-3259

Health First Leeza's Place
3661 Babcock Street,
Melbourne, Fl 32901
Telephone: (321) 951-7118
Fax: (321) 951-7280

Leeza's Place at Memorial Hospital Pembroke
2261 N. University Drive, Suite 103
Pembroke Pines, FL 33024
Telephone: (954) 967-7240
Fax: (954) 967-7241

Leeza's Place at Provena Saint Joseph Medical Center
113 Republic Avenue
Joliet, IL 60435
Telephone: (815) 741-0077
Fax: (815) 741-7069
Leeza's Place at WellMed
14100 Nacogdoches Rd, #120

San Antonio, TX 78247
Telephone: 210) 599-4614
Fax: (210) 599-4093

Leeza's Place by WellMed
at the Bob Ross Senior Center
2219 Babcock Road
San Antonio, TX 78222
Telephone: 210) 207-5310
Fax: (210) 589-6539

Leeza's Place by WellMed
In Lower Rio Grande Valley
5401 S. McColl Road
Edinburg, TX 78539
Telephone: 956-566-2671

Leeza's Place at GLEH
1602 N. Ivar Avenue
Hollywood, CA 90028

National Alliance for Caregiving
4720 Montgomery Lane, 5th Floor
Bethesda, MD 20814
Email: info@caregiving.org
Website: http://www.caregiving.org/
Provides support to family caregivers and the professionals
who help them and raises public awareness of issues facing family
caregivers.

National Caregivers Library
901 Moorefield Park Drive Suite 100
Richmond, VA 23236
Telephone: (804) 327-1112
Website: http://www.caregiverslibrary.org/
An extensive online library for caregivers.

The National Family Caregivers Association
10400 Connecticut Avenue, Suite 500
Kensington, MD 20895-3944
Telephone: (800) 896-3650
Fax: (301) 942-2302
Email: info@thefamilycaregiver.org
http://www.thefamilycaregiver.org/about_nfca/
Educates, supports, empowers and advocates for the more than 50 million Americans who care for loved ones with a chronic illness or disability or the frailties of old age.

Physicians, Hospitals, and Clinics

The AGS Foundation for Health in Aging
  (American Geriatrics Society)
Empire State Building
350 Fifth Avenue, Suite 801
New York, New York 10118
Telephone: (800) 563-4916
Fax: (212) 832-8646
Website: www.healthinaging.org
Provides a physician referral service at no charge. All physicians participating in the referral service are members of the American Geriatrics Society.

Health Resources and Services Administration – Bureau of Primary Health Care

Website: http://www.bphc.hrsa.gov/

Helps you find a clinic for medical care, even if you have no medical insurance.

Medline Plus

Website: http://www.nlm.nih.gov/medlineplus/directories.html

Online resource for finding health professionals and facilities

Revolution Health

1250 Connecticut Avenue NW, Ste. 600

Washington, DC 20036-2651

Email: customercare@revolutionhealth.com

Website: http://www.revolutionhealth.com/care-providers

Assists in locating health professionals and facilities.

Veterans Health Administration

VA Benefits: (800) 827-1000

Health Care Benefits: (877) 222-8387

Website: http://www1.va.gov/directory/guide/home.asp

Serves the needs of America's veterans by providing primary care, specialized care, and related medical and social support services.

Government and Social Service Agencies

Administration on Aging

Washington, DC 20201

Telephone: (202) 619-0724

Fax: (202) 357-3555

E-mail: aoainfo@aoa.hhs.gov

Eldercare Locator (to find services for an older person in his or her locality): (800) 677-1116

Website: http://www.aoa.gov/about/contact/contact.asp

AoA is one of the nation's largest providers of home and community-based care for older persons and their caregivers.

U.S. Department of Health and Human Services

200 Independence Avenue, S.W.

Washington, D.C. 20201

Telephone: (877) 696-6775

Website: http://www.hhs.gov/

The principal federal agency charged with protecting the health of all Americans and providing essential human services, especially for those who are least able to help themselves.

DisabilityInfo.gov

Website: http://www.disabilityinfo.gov

A comprehensive online resource designed to provide people with disabilities with quick and easy access to the information they need on numerous subjects, including benefits, civil rights, community life, education, employment, housing, health, technology and transportation.

Food and Drug Administration

5600 Fishers Lane

Rockville, MD 20857-0001

Telephone: (888) INFO-FDA

Website: http://www.fda.gov

The FDA regulates the nation's drug industry. It maintains

information on all drugs and treatments that are available to consumers in the United States.

National Institute on Aging
Building 31, Room 5C27
31 Center Drive, MSC 2292
Bethesda, MD 20892
Phone: (301) 496-1752
Fax: (301) 496-1072
Website: http://www.nia.nih.gov
NIA is an arm of the National Institutes of Health and leads the federal government's efforts in aging research.

National Institutes of Health
9000 Rockville Pike
Bethesda, Maryland 20894
Telephone: (301) 496-4000
Email: NIHinfo@od.nih.gov
Website: http://www.nih.gov
The primary federal agency for conducting and supporting medical research.

Office of Special Education and Rehabilitative Services
U.S. Department of Education
400 Maryland Ave., S.W.
Washington, DC 20202-7100
Telephone: (202) 245-7468
Website: http://www.ed.gov/about/offices/list/osers/
An office committed to improving outcomes for people with disabilities of all ages.

Health Insurance

Benefits Checkup
Website: http://www.benefitscheckup.org/
A service of the National Council on Aging, Benefits Checkup is an online resource that helps people connect to private or government programs.

Medicare
Website: www.Medicare.gov
The website provides assistance and information on financial benefits for health care that you may be entitled to.

Hospice and Palliative Care Organizations

The Five Wishes
Website: http://www.agingwithdignity.org/5wishes.html
Helps you express how you want to be treated if you are seriously ill and unable to speak for yourself.

Caring Connections
HelpLine: (800) 658-8898
Multilingual Line: (877) 658-8896
Email: caringinfo@nhpco.org
Website: http://www.caringinfo.org/
Information on palliative care and end of life issues.

Center to Advance Palliative Care
The Center to Advance Palliative Care
1255 Fifth Avenue, Suite C-2
New York, NY 10029

Telephone: (212) 201-2670

http://www.capc.org/

Provides health care professionals with the tools, training and technical assistance necessary to start and sustain successful palliative care programs in hospitals and other health care settings.

Growth House, Inc.

http://www.growthhouse.org/

An internet search portal to resources for life-threatening illness and end of life care.

Hospice and Palliative Care Association of New York State

21 Aviation Road, Suite 9

Albany, NY 12205

Telephone: (518) 446-1483

Fax: (518) 446-1484

Website: http://www.hpcanys.org/about_hp.asp

A not-for-profit organization representing hospice and palliative care programs, allied organizations and individuals interested in the development and growth of quality, comprehensive end-of-life services.

National Hospice and Palliative Care Organization

1700 Diagonal Road, Suite 625

Alexandria, Virginia 22314

Telephone: (703) 837-1500

Fax: (703) 837-1233

HelpLine: (800) 568-8898

Website: http://www.nhpco.org/templates/1/homepage.cfm

A resource on many caregiving issues for those individuals and families facing serious illness.

Medical Professional Associations

American Academy of Family Physicians
11400 Tomahawk Creek Parkway
Leawood, KS 66211-2672
Telephone: (800) 274-2237 / (913) 906-6000
Fax: (913) 906-6075
Website: http://www.familydoctor.org
Provides a listing of physicians specializing in family medicine.

American Academy of Neurology
1080 Montreal Avenue
Saint Paul, MN 55116
Telephone: (800) 879-1960 / (651) 695-2717
Fax: (651) 695-2791
Website: http://www.aan.com/go/public
Provides a listing of physicians specializing in neurological care.

American Geriatrics Society
The Empire State Building
350 Fifth Avenue, Suite 801
New York, NY 10118
Telephone: (212) 308-1414
Email: info@americangeriatrics.org
Website: http://www.americangeriatrics.org
A not-for-profit organization of 7,000 health professionals devoted to improving the health, independence and quality of life of all older people.

Other Non-Profit Resources

American Association of Retired Persons

601 E Street NW

Washington, DC 20049

Telephone: (202) 434-2277 / (888) 687-2277

Website: http://www.aarp.org/

A good source for long-term care options, caregiving, legal and financial planning, Medicare and Medicaid information and legislative issues affecting the elderly.

ARCH National Respite Network

800 Eastowne Drive, Suite 105

Chapel Hill, North Carolina 27514

Telephone: (919) 490-5577

Fax: (919) 490-4905

Website: http://chtop.org/ARCH.html

Information on temporary relief for caregivers and families who are caring for those with disabilities, chronic or terminal illnesses, or the elderly.

Catholic Charities USA

Sixty-Six Canal Center Plaza, Suite 600

Alexandria, Virginia 22314

Telephone: (703) 549-1390

Fax: (703) 549-1656

Website: http://www.catholiccharitiesusa.org/

Catholic Charities agencies and institutions nationwide provide vital social services to people in need, regardless of their religious, social, or economic backgrounds.

Jewish Board of Family and Children's Services
120 West 57th Street
New York, NY 10019
Telephone: (212) 582-9100 / (888) 523-2769
Website: http://www.jbfcs.org/
Serves over 65,000 New Yorkers annually from all religious, ethnic, and economic backgrounds through community-based programs, residential facilities, and day-treatment centers.

National Alliance for Hispanic Health
1501 Sixteenth Street, NW
Washington, DC 20036
Telephone: (202) 387-5000
Website: http://www.hispanichealth.org/
The premier organization focusing on Hispanic health. Reaches over 14 million Hispanic consumers throughout the U.S.

Volunteers of America
1660 Duke Street
Alexandria, VA 22314
Telephone: (703) 341-5000
Fax: (703) 341-7000
Website: http://www.voa.org/
A major provider of professional long-term nursing care for seniors and others coping with illness or injury. They offer a continuum of services that includes assisted living, memory care, nursing care, rehabilitative therapy, and more.

Online Resources

Today's Caregiver

http://www.caregiver.com

Together with Today's Caregiver magazine, the first national magazine dedicated to caregivers, the "Sharing Wisdom Caregivers Conferences", caregiver.com provides topic-specific newsletters, online discussion lists, back issue articles of Today's Caregiver magazine, chat rooms and an online store, the Fearless Caregiver book, regional Fearless Caregiver conferences and the annual Caregiver Friendly awards program. Caregiver Media Group and all of its products are developed for caregivers, about caregivers and by caregivers.

Caring Today

http://www.caringtoday.com

Since 2004, Caring Today has addressed the needs of America's 50 million caregivers with expertise, understanding and answers through its quarterly national magazine and this website, as well as e-newsletters and custom-publishing projects. Caring Today magazine reaches two million people who turn to it for relief from day-to-day stress, support from other caregivers, advice from experts in a wide variety of relevant fields, resources to assist you, and answers to your questions.

The Alzheimer's Store

http://www.alzstore.com

The Alzheimer's Store is dedicated to providing unique products and information for those caring for someone with Alzheimer's disease. Every product in the store has been carefully selected to make living with Alzheimer's disease as easy as possible.

CareCentral
1655 N Fort Myer Drive, Suite 400
Arlington, VA 22209
Telephone: (703) 302-1040
Fax: (703) 248-0830
Website: http://www.carecentral.com/
CareCentral allows you or your loved one to create your own personalized website to provide friends and families with a central hub to keep in touch, stay informed, and share support.

CaringBridge
1995 Rahn Cliff Court, Suite 200
Eagan, MN 55122
Telephone: (651) 452-7940
Website: http://www.caringbridge.org/
Offers free personalized websites to those wishing to stay in touch with family and friends during significant life events.

Lotsa Helping Hands
365 Boston Post Road, Suite 157
Sudbury, MA 01776
Email: information@lotsahelpinghands.com
Website: http://www.lotsahelpinghands.com
Provides online an easy-to-use, private group calendar, specifically designed for organizing helpers, where everyone can pitch in with meals delivery, rides, and other tasks necessary for life to run smoothly during a crisis.

Scrapbooking, Stamping, and Other Creative Activities

If you'd like to exchange ideas with other scrapbook, stamping and home craft enthusiasts, there are many forums online. For example, try accessing the groups at Yahoo.com. Simply open Yahoo.com, click on Groups, and enter your area of interest.

BOOKS ON SCRAPBOOKING:

Scrapbook Page Maps: Sketches for Creative Layouts, by Becky Fleck, F & W Publications, 2008.

The Amazing Page: 650 Scrapbook Page Ideas, Tips and Techniques, by Memory Makers Books, 2006

Encyclopedia of Scrapbooking, by Creative Keepsakes, Sunset Publishing, 2005.

BOOKS ON STAMPING:

Texture Effects for Rubber Stamping, by Nancy Curry, F & W Publications, 2004

The Rubber Stamper's Bible, by Francoise Reid, F & W Publications, 2005

Appendix

If you are a caregiver, you're in good company! There are literally tens of millions of caregivers, and almost nine million of them care for someone 50 years of age or older with a memory loss disorder. The majority of individuals reading this book are most likely primary caregivers. These are the caregivers who provide the primary support, often around the clock, needed by patients who are suffering from chronic illnesses, and in the case of this book, memory disorders. But some caregivers face special challenges due to their age, ethnic or cultural background, relationship to the loved one, gender or other reason. These special situations require additional or different strategies and techniques for ensuring the caregiver's health and happiness. There is one thing, however, that all caregivers share. It's the need to *Take Your Oxygen First!* Here we will explore some of these groups of caregivers and their unique circumstances, and offer some solutions that address their special needs.

THE SANDWICH GENERATION

An estimated 5.7 million Americans both care for aging relatives and have children for whom they care. These so-called "sandwich generation" caregivers make up forty-one percent of the caregiver population. Nearly two-thirds have said they lack enough information about how to help their children cope when a loved one is diagnosed with Alzheimer's disease, and "sandwich caregivers" can find themselves pushed and pulled from two directions as they give care to their memory impaired loved one while also looking after the needs of their children. But there are encouraging developments. A majority of sandwich caregivers report that their children are assisting them in giving care to their loved ones, often performing tasks such as helping with dressing, feeding and transportation, and most of those who feel they are doing well with their caregiving roles attribute this success in part to the assistance they're receiving from the younger members of the family.

Oxygen For Sandwich Generation Caregivers

- Heed the advice of this book: keep your physical and emotionalspiritual health in top shape.
- Carefully plan to address the impact your caregiving duties will have on the generations that depend on you.
- Plan ahead and try to keep organized. Organize activities such as those detailed in Chapter 10 of this book for everyone.
- Explore options for respite for both age groups.
- Have a backup plan for caregiving for both groups.
- Be accepting of offers of help.
- Take steps to ensure the younger generation has adequate support for understanding the illness and the impact on their own lives.

EMPLOYED CAREGIVERS

The majority of adult caregivers are employed. Among baby boomer caregivers (aged 50-64 years), almost two thirds are working full or part time while providing care for a loved one 18 to 40 hours a month. The impact of this time spent in caregiving is profound, to the worker and to the workplace. Employed caregivers frequently lose a great deal of earning potential over time. They also have to rearrange their schedules frequently, which can cause problems not only for themselves but can create tension and disruption at work. Female caregivers are often affected more severely, since statistically they are likely to spend twelve years out of the workforce raising children and caring for a relative. This can have serious consequences for a female caregiver's financial security in her later years.

Oxygen For The Employed Caregiver

- Take Your Oxygen First: keep your physical, emotional and spiritual health in top shape.
- Have a system of care in place to allow you to manage both your workplace responsibilities and your caregiving responsibilities: backup caregiving, care managers, internet based cameras, private duty companionship are all options you should consider.
- Investigate "eldercare assistance" as part of your workplace benefit package. These assistance programs include informatio and referral to services and programs that can help you care for your loved one. *Working Mother Magazine* conducts an annual survey of good workplaces for women. Check out the survey for those with programs supporting caregivers. www.workingmother.com Talk to your Human Resources department if your company hasn't jumped on the bandwagon!

LONG DISTANCE CAREGIVERS

Long distance caregivers are just that. They are loved ones who, for whatever reason: geographic, emotional or vocational, cannot be present on a day-to-day basis with their loved one. Statistically, if you're a long distance caregiver you are one of the up to seven million caregivers who live more than an hour from the person in your care. Regardless of the time you spend in your caregiving commute, you are very prone to additional stress and anxiety.

In some cases the long-distance caregiver is the primary caregiver as well. If that's you, creating on-site care teams from among other family members, friends, and paid caregivers is critical.

If you are a long distance caregiver but not a primary caregiver, your input can be valuable, but be respectful of the feelings of the primary caregiver, and keep your involvement consistent. Nothing is more damaging to the spirit of a primary caregiver than to have a long-distance caregiver arrive for the holidays, proclaim everything a "mess", and then return to their home without offering assistance!

Oxygen For Long-distance Caregivers

If You are Both a Long-Distance and Primary Caregiver:

- Take Your Oxygen First: keep your physical, emotional and spiritual health in top shape.
- Find a local resource person. This is your "go to" person. He or she might be an extended family member or friend who is familiar with local resources.
- Consider hiring a care manager (for older adults, a geriatric care manager). Find one at www.caremanagers.org.
- Develop a two-tier backup plan for caregiving responsibilities. Due to the unpredictable nature of caregiving for someone with a memory loss disorder, it helps to have more than one set of people to step in if you are unable to provide care.
- Accept offers of help from neighbors, church members, and others.
- Establish a good rapport with your loved one's primary physician and get cleared to communicate directly with his or her

office about your loved one's care.

- Carefully and proactively plan for the "long haul." Have a one, three and five-year plan for your loved one's needs and for your own.

If You are a Long-distance Caregiver but Not the Primary Caregiver:

- All of the above and
- Offer to provide respite for the primary caregiver. Plan either a one or two-week stay with your loved one or pay for a good long respite for the primary caregiver.
- Ask frequently about the finances and do your share of the work in making sure that expenses are taken care of.

SENIOR CAREGIVERS

Many senior caregivers rank their own health and quality of life as poor—even after the person in their care moves to a facility or passes on. The mortality rate for elderly caregivers is higher than for non-caregiving seniors of the same age. Seniors face unique pressures as caregivers. For some, the transition to being caregiver is a natural and easy one. For others, it is terribly difficult. There are feelings of loss and sadness, or perhaps anger and resentment, as the illness robs the caregiver and her loved one of their golden years together. At Leeza's Place we offer lecture series and other caregiver training and support programs to help caregivers work through the emotions and learn the skills they need in this new role. The Alzheimer's Association has numerous resources available in most areas for caregiver training and support which can be found online at www.alz.org.

Oxygen For Senior Caregivers

- Take Your Oxygen First: keep your physical, emotional and spiritual health in top shape.
- Become knowledgeable of resources for respite in your community. Schedule a regular day of respite each week and one week per year at a minimum.
- Have a backup plan for caregiving ready to go if you should become ill or need medical testing or hospitalization.
- Be accepting of offers of help.
- Consider in-home personal response units to summon emergency personnel if needed.
- Consider getting a medical alert bracelet identifying your loved one's disorder and identifying you as a caregiver of someone with a memory loss disorder.

HUSBANDS AND SONS AS CAREGIVERS

Much like nursing, caregiving has often been considered a woman's job. The skills required for caregiving, including grooming, cooking, cleaning and some aspects of personal care for another are often quite new to a husband or son. Some men never become comfortable with providing certain aspects of personal care, but paid caregivers can be hired to supplement care.

Many men have been reared to avoid asking for help. That means they are less likely to reach out to friends and family or to social service agencies. Men are also less open with their feelings. The caregiving process is a tidal wave of emotions, including some that may be completely new to the male caregiver. Male caregivers need outlets for the emotional stresses they experience during caregiving. At Leeza's Place we have caregiver training and support programs that address the needs of both male and female caregivers. Just like the ladies, the husbands and sons need to take the oxygen first.

Oxygen For Husbands And Sons As Caregivers

- Take Your Oxygen First: keep your physical, emotional and spiritual health in top shape.
- Learn about resources for respite in your community. Schedule a regular day of respite each week and one week per year at a minimum.
- Get help when your loved one needs help in the bathroom. Often this can be a good place to begin using a paid caregiver.
- Have a backup plan for caregiving ready if you should become ill or need medical testing or hospitalization.
- Be accepting of offers of help.
- Consider in-home personal response units to summon emergency personnel if needed.
- Consider acquiring a medical alert bracelet identifying your loved one's disorder and identifying you as a caregiver.

STEP FAMILIES

In addition to all the usual challenges discussed above, families created by remarriage can face unique issues when one of the couple falls ill. When both husband and wife have children from a first marriage, it is critical that the children develop strong relationships so they can work well together when needed. Depending on the financial and legal arrangements set up at the time of the marriage, there can be problems paying for care. While the exact circumstances vary widely, it's critical for families to clearly discuss the wishes of the couple ahead of time. Durable powers of attorney need to be created. If there are long-distance issues and primary caregiving issues, those need to be addressed well ahead of time.

Oxygen For Step Family Caregivers

- Follow the advice in this book and Take Your Oxygen First.
- Respect the family bonds. If you are a stepchild, refrain from rendering your opinion unless directly asked.
- Communicate early and often with your siblings, be they full siblings or step-siblings.
- Determine with as much detail as possible the financial arrangements for providing care.

SIBLINGS

Sibling groups participating in giving care have more talent and manpower to draw upon, but also have to deal with multiple sets of feelings, relationships, and life circumstances while attending to the needs of their loved one. They will have their own mix of talents, personal preferences, and limitations due to geography or personal choice. Spend time talking about how each sibling can contribute to the overall care needs.

Oxygen For Sibling Caregivers

- Take Your Oxygen First—*all* of you!
- Remember that birth order doesn't need to dictate the caregiving roles. Be honest about your potential contributions.
- Communicate frequently.
- Provide respite for each other.

YOUNG AND NEXT GENERATION CAREGIVERS

It is very important that we reach out to children who are dealing with the chronic illness of someone they love. Being a parent or grandparent of a child caregiver requires us to be very vigilant in being fair, consistent and available to the child while making sure that the process is enriching and not depleting for the younger person.

In addition to feeling overwhelmed by their own roles within the caregiving process, children can also become afraid that their loved one's memory disorder may eventually claim them. They are often faced with the concept mortality long before they are emotionally ready for it. If you are a young member of a family in which care is being given to someone older, you can be a great help. More and more young people like you are embracing the challenge, and the potential joy, of making caregiving a family affair.

Oxygen For Young Caregivers

- Communicate frequently with your parents about the illness. Keep the lines of communication open at all times. Encourage them to share with you both the good and the bad. Learn along with your parents about the illness. Ask them if there are websites or books where you can read about it.
- Figure out how you can best participate in the caregiving process. Can you take over for your mom so that she can get to her own doctor's appointment or go play a round of golf? Can you do the grocery shopping or two loads of laundry to ease the burden back home?

AFRICAN-AMERICAN CAREGIVERS

Among different ethnic groups, the caregiving process can involve family members in a variety of ways distinct to their ethnicity. In African-American communities, the family members are more likely to care at home for elders with dementia, and usually seek support from other family members rather than from outside agencies. Despite this tendency to keep the process at home, African-American caregivers report fewer burdens than average, perhaps because of coping skills that include a strong faith in God and the ability to adapt to adverse circumstances. Harnessing the power of extended family networks is also beneficial to African-American caregivers, as it is to other cultures and families that embrace it.

Oxygen For African-American Caregivers

- Take Your Oxygen First: keep your physical, emotional and spiritual health in top shape.
- If you will be caring for your loved one at home, remember that you need to have respite from your caregiving responsibilities at times. Look to your local faith-based or civic community centers for support. Learn about local resources for respite care. Encourage your siblings or other long-distance caregivers to help give you a break.
- Develop a two-tier backup plan for caregiving responsibilities. Due to the unpredictable nature of caregiving for someone with a memory loss disorder, it helps to have more than one set of people to step in if you are unable to provide care.
- Accept offers of help from within and outside of the family.
- Carefully and proactively plan for the "long haul". Have a one, three and five-year plan for your loved one's needs and for your own.

HISPANIC CAREGIVERS

Over the next two decades, the Hispanic population in the United States is expected to grow by over 1.2 million annually. The Leeza Gibbons Memory Foundation and every other organization that wants to stay ahead in the world of caregiving are dedicating vital resources to meet the needs of caregivers within the Hispanic community.

Traditionally, Hispanics have maintained close, supportive ties to their family members, even to those outside the immediate family that live in the same home. Hispanic women have traditionally assumed the role of primary caregiver for chronically ill elderly relatives. More than with other groups, Hispanic caregivers report that they are especially burdened by the shame of behavioral and cognitive changes in their loved one. This makes it difficult for them to reach out and share embarrassing situations about a family member's medical condition with strangers, healthcare professionals, and community service agencies.

Oxygen For Hispanic Caregivers

- Take Your Oxygen First: keep your physical, emotional and spiritual health in top shape.
- If you will be caring for your loved one at home, remember that you still need to have respite from your caregiving responsibilities at times. Look to your local faith-based or civic community centers for support. Learn about local resources for respite care. Encourage your siblings or other long-distance caregivers to give you a break.
- Develop a two-tier backup plan for caregiving responsibilities. Due to the unpredictable nature of caregiving for some-

one with a memory loss disorder, it helps to have more than one set of people to step in if you are unable to provide care.

■ Accept offers of help from within and outside of the family.

■ Carefully and proactively plan for the "long haul." Have a one, three and five-year plan in place for your loved one's needs and for your own.

GAY AND LESBIAN CAREGIVERS

Gay and lesbian caregivers have all of the psychological challenges that any primary caregiver has, but their sexual orientation can bring additional complications. While government agencies, non-profit organizations and the media have finally begun to focus on the needs of seniors and caregivers, less attention has been given to the needs of this group. There are still many societal barriers to the gay caregivers' need for education, empowerment and energy. These barriers exist as well for gay care *receivers*, and it's not unusual for individuals who have "come out" and become comfortable with their sexuality to have to "go back to the closet" when placed in a residential care facility. Increased acceptance of the gay lifestyle in the past two decades has prompted a greater awareness among social service providers nationwide about the gay community, especially in major urban centers. Depending on where you live and what kind of support or prejudice you've experienced in the past, you may feel reluctant discussing issues related to sexual orientation when dealing with government and private agencies. Whether the person for whom you care is a parent, partner or friend, you will find it easiest to get answers or act as an advocate with public agencies, community nonprofits and hospitals if your loved one has legally designated you to act on his or her behalf. Gay caregivers may find that they have less support than they would like from their own—or their care receiver's—biological family members. If this is true in your situation, developing a support system comprised of trusted friends and sensitive community services and programs will be especially important.

Oxygen For Gay And Lesbian Caregivers

- Take Your Oxygen First: keep your physical, emotional and spiritual health in top shape.
- Learn about local resources for respite care. Encourage your siblings or other long-distance caregivers to give you a break.
- Develop a two-tier backup plan for caregiving responsibilities. Due to the unpredictable nature of caregiving for someone with a memory loss disorder, it helps to have more than one set of people to step in if you are unable to provide care.
- Accept offers of help from within and outside of the family.
- Carefully and proactively plan for the "long haul." Have a one, three and five-year plan in place for your loved one's needs and for your own.

ABOUT THE AUTHORS

Leeza Gibbons

She has been called a social entrepreneur, but if you ask Leeza Gibbons what she does, she'll simply answer "I'm a story teller". From television news journalist and host to radio personality, producer and businesswoman, Gibbons has been entering America's living rooms for almost 30 years. She currently hosts and produces the internationally syndicated radio program *Hollywood Confidential*, but she first burst on the national scene as an anchor and reporter on *Entertainment Tonight*. It wouldn't be until hosting her own daytime talk show, *Leeza*, that audiences would see Gibbons' determination to get outside the box and become a household name while highlighting her intelligence, sensitivity and compassion.

Gibbons has a star on Hollywood's fabled Walk of Fame, but she will tell you she is most proud of being a mom to "three of the planet's most amazing kids." Two of them grew up on the Paramount lot where she served as the host and executive producer of Leeza, which aired from 1994 to 2000 and which garnered 27 Emmy Award nominations. Gibbons went on to become the managing editor and host of the television newsmagazine *EXTRA* until she left in 2002 to form her nonprofit organization, The Leeza Gibbons Memory Foundation and its signature program, Leeza's Place. Leeza and her family, together with co-founder James Huysman, created the Foundation in tribute to Leeza's mother and grandmother, both of whom died of Alzheimer's disease, and in response to the growing needs of those who suffer from disease and chronic illness and their caregivers.

James Huysman, PsyD, LCSW

Dr. Huysman is the co-founder and Executive Director of the Leeza Gibbons Memory Foundation, a non-profit organization dedicated to the education, empowerment and energizing of caregivers and their family members who deal daily with family members who suffer from long-term chronic disorders. He is a psychologist, board certified therapist in clinical social work, crisis interventionist, certified addictions professional and a certified compassion fatigue therapist. The recipient of a PsyD in psychology from Cal Southern University and a Master's degree in social work from Barry University, he has developed national behavioral health programs, served as on and off-camera clinical consultant to scores of national television programs, and served as a corporate officer for a number of hospitals and independent psychiatric and addiction centers nationwide.

Rosemary DeAngelis Laird, M.D.

Dr. Laird is the founding Medical Director of the Health First Aging Institute located in Melbourne, Florida. Established in 2002, the Aging Institute sponsors clinics for geriatric consultation, memory loss and primary care, and educational and support programs for caregivers. Dr. Laird received her medical degree from Georgetown University School of Medicine and completed residency training in Internal Medicine at the University of Chicago. She completed a Geriatric Fellowship and received a Master's degree in Health Services Administration from the University of Kansas.

Index